ULTIMATE OLYMPIC WEIGHTLIFTING

A Complete Guide from Beginning to Gold Medal

DAVE RANDOLPH

Published in the United States by
Ulysses Press
P.O. Box 3440
Berkeley, CA 94703
www.ulyssespress.com

ISBN: 978-1-61243-445-2
Library of Congress Control Number: 2014952017

Printed in the United States
10 9 8 7 6 5 4 3 2 1

Acquisitions: Katherine Furman
Managing editor: Claire Chun
Editor: Lily Chou
Proofreader: Lauren Harrison
Indexer: Sayre Van Young
Front cover design: what!design @ whatweb.com
Front cover photographs: studio © Petrenko Andriy/shutterstock.com
Models: Tyler Agajan, April Gemein, Dave Randolph
Makeup: Sabrina Foster/sabrinafostermakeup.com

CONTENTS

PART 1
OVERVIEW

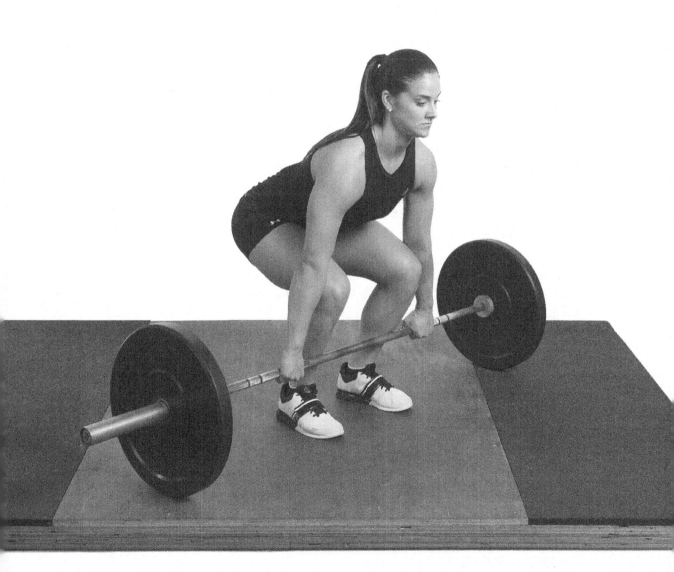

INTRODUCTION

Olympic weightlifting (using a barbell and plates to get a weight overhead) has been around since the mid- to late 1800s. However, it wasn't until the late 1940s and 1950s that the sport transformed into the Olympic lifting practiced today—the "clean and jerk" and the "snatch."

Up until fairly recently, most people had no idea what Olympic weightlifting is. Maybe they caught a lift watching the Olympic Games or on ABC's *Wide World of Sports*. The pool of those who actually wanted to learn the lifts wasn't very big, either, and those who did want to learn had even fewer qualified coaches nearby.

This all changed when CrossFit hit the scene in 2000. Because of this incredibly popular exercise craze, which features the clean and jerk and snatch in its varied routines, these old-school movements are becoming mainstream ways to stay fit and healthy. Now everyone has not only heard of the lifts and seen them done, but has probably tried them as well. I wrote this book to be a concise course in learning the Olympic lifts. While the lifts require a lot of work to achieve a high level of proficiency, you don't need to be an Olympic-caliber lifter to reap the benefits.

In this book you'll learn the proper way to execute the lifts by breaking each one into easily learnable chunks. Once you master the basic components and refine your technique over the weeks, the pieces will start to come together.

Also included are general nutrition guidelines for eating properly, an important factor for optimal performance when lifting and for overall health. In addition, the essential self-assessment section will identify areas that need strengthening, followed by targeted exercise fixes to address those weaknesses. (Remember: Injuries are not necessarily caused by technique issues, but poor technique will break you.) A 12-week program, broken into three 4-week phases, guides you from raw beginner to proficient weightlifter.

Olympic weightlifting, along with a clean diet, will make you athletic, powerful, and lean. By incorporating mobility and agility work, you'll be able to do pretty much any everyday activity without difficulty.

WHY OLYMPIC WEIGHTLIFTING?

If you're looking for a quick fix or are hoping to perfect your movement in a short period of time, Olympic weightlifting is not for you. But if you want to develop explosive strength and incredible athleticism, Olympic weightlifting will help you achieve these goals. Be forewarned: You'll need to put in the time. To be really good at the sport, even if you never plan to compete, takes a lot of practice using low reps and a lot of sets.

A lot of gyms use high-rep Olympic lifts because they're metabolically demanding, meaning they require a lot of energy and therefore will make you lose weight. In many cases it's quantity over quality, and therein lies the problem. Unfortunately, even with a light weight, doing 20 or 30 reps of cleans pushes the envelope of safety. Sure, you should push yourself to the point of fatigue, but you also need to know when enough is enough. Listen to your body, not your head. You have to know your limits.

With that said, practicing Olympic weightlifting will help you lose weight by increasing energy expenditure and by building dense muscle mass. However, you won't look like a bodybuilder. Bodybuilding, or hypertrophy training, is quite a bit different from Olympic weightlifting. Unlike snatches and clean and jerks, bodybuilding movements focus more on body parts rather than the whole body. While bodybuilding focuses on making your muscles bigger and stronger, Olympic weightlifting will help you get lean and athletic in both appearance and quality of movement.

Olympic weightlifting is very challenging and technical. The top lifters have been training for years. Just like any other sport, being a skilled lifter means lots of high-quality practice along with a coach who knows how to create programs and to perfect the nuances required to reach the upper levels of Olympic weightlifting. Whether you're just starting out or have been lifting for a while, this book will help guide you on your path to a stronger and better you.

HISTORY OF OLYMPIC WEIGHTLIFTING

Man has been lifting heavy stuff in some form or another since the dawn of time. It probably didn't take long for two guys to get together to see who could lift the heaviest rock. In the Middle Ages, men fashioned their own "dumb-bells," so called because the clappers were removed from actual church bells so they wouldn't make noise while being lifted. In ancient Greece, where the Olympics began, there are all sorts of images depicting weightlifting challenges. The sport itself initially appeared in the 1896 Olympics, but the first crowning of a champion was actually in 1891. Of course, the implements used in the 1800s were a far cry from today's high-tech bars and rubber bumper plates.

THE CHANGING FACE OF OLYMPIC LIFTS

The early Olympic lifts themselves were quite a bit different than they are today. Originally, the lifters competed in a one-arm lift and a two-arm lift. After its initial inception in 1896, the sport was dropped from the 1900 Games, returned in 1904, then eliminated again until after World War I.

In the 1920 Games held in Antwerp, Belgium, Olympic weightlifting returned. The lifts at the time were the one-handed "snatch" and one- and two-handed "clean and jerks." Two more lifts—the two-handed snatch and the two-handed press—were added in the 1924 Games. The Olympic sport continued to be fine-tuned over the years, with lifts added then removed. In 1928, the one-handed lifts were dropped. In the name of fairness, weight classes were added in 1932 so you no longer had a 300-pound participant competing against a 150-pound lifter.

In the 1950s, the deadlift, bench press, and squat (lifts now considered "power lifts") were also contested in Olympic weightlifting. All three were dropped and then reclassified under a new sport called "powerlifting."

Due to the ease of "cheating," the clean and press lift was dropped from the sport after the 1972 Olympics. Basically, you could lean backward and almost make it a bench press, so the various Olympic-lifting organizations decided to remove the clean and press from the sport. In a nod to gender equality, the 2000 Sydney Olympics featured women's Olympic weightlifting for the first time.

EVOLVING TECHNIQUES

Throughout the 20th century the technique of the primary lifts changed as people found what worked best for getting heavy weight overhead. But while the snatch, clean and jerk, and military press were evolving on the Olympic front, many countries continued to train and compete with their own versions of lifts and equipment. The Russians favored high-repetition kettlebell lifting, which became a true sport in the 1970s and '80s. Other countries lifted heavy stones to shoulder height. Other lifts were dropped over time, but today there are two primary lifts in competition: the barbell snatch and the barbell clean and jerk.

As in any sport, there are lots of variations in program design. But despite previous regional differences, teaching methodologies are now fairly standard. The snatch and the clean and jerk are commonplace and are easier than ever to learn and integrate into your workout routine.

WHAT IS OLYMPIC WEIGHTLIFTING?

Some form of Olympic weightlifting has been around since the 19th century. Through decades of evolution, today the Olympic lifts are officially two moves: the "clean and jerk" and the "snatch."

Please note that "lifting weights" and "weightlifting" are *not* the same thing. The former refers to lifting any sort of weight—barbells, dumbbells, rocks, kettlebells, etc. The latter refers specifically to the two modern-day Olympic lifts: the snatch and the clean and jerk.

In the snatch, the weight is brought from the ground to overhead using two hands and is locked out overhead in one smooth movement while simultaneously dropping into a rock-bottom squat. The clean portion of the clean and jerk involves bringing the weight (these days a barbell or kettlebell) to shoulder level, called the "rack position." The jerk portion involves quickly dropping under the bar while simultaneously straightening out the arms until the elbows are locked, then standing up with the weight overhead. However, this isn't a pressing action—that's quite different.

There are many variations of these two lifts. They're used to not only teach the full lifts but to allow almost anyone to train and perfect some aspect of the lifts. A lot of people split the clean and jerk into two separate exercises; this is fine on a technical training level, but you can't compete in clean only or jerk only.

The primary movement called the clean begins with a barbell on the floor over the middle portion of the feet. You assume a semi-squat/hip-hinge position and explosively stand up, driving the hips forward and pulling hard with the arms. As the bar goes up, momentum kicks in; as the bar approaches the level of the solar plexus, you quickly drop into a deep squat while dropping the elbows under the bar, rotating them forward, and "catching" the bar on the front of the shoulders with the fingers of each hand holding the bar in place.

After completing the clean, you stand up, maintaining the bar in the "rack" position across the front of the shoulders. Once standing, you'll quickly drop under the bar, landing in a split stance while simultaneously straightening out the arms so the bar goes overhead. *Note:* This is not a press. You're literally moving under the bar as it rises, with your hands remaining almost at the same height they were at the start of the jerk. The arms straighten as the body is lowered.

Once the bar is caught overhead, you must keep it overhead while returning to a standing position. You must be totally locked out and stable for the lift to count. In competitions, the bar is dropped to the floor in a controlled manner, which is why bumper plates are used. For everyday Olympic weightlifting, you'll want to return the bar to rack then drop it in front of you while squatting it to the floor. This will keep your equipment from getting torn up or damaging the floor.

Snatches also start with the bar on the floor in the same position as the clean. The spacing of the hands on the bar is quite a bit wider when doing snatches—this makes the lift a little easier and more forgiving on shoulders that may not have full range of motion or for those with a tight upper back. Like the clean, the snatch starts off very explosively but, as the bar moves up, it goes all the way overhead. As the bar reaches mid-torso level, you drop into a deep squat, catching the bar overhead. From here, you stand up with full control of the bar, elbows and knees locked out, and absolutely no movement. Once the judges give a go or no-go, you'll return the bar to the floor, ending the lift.

Outside of Olympic competition you'll find variations of these two lifts, including "assistance" lifts designed to help the lifter focus on a specific portion of the movement. Other modified exercises allow lifters with limited mobility to perform the lifts. For example, the "clean" portion of the clean and jerk requires a tremendous amount of hip and ankle flexibility, something most people don't possess due to a sedentary lifestyle. So the lifter does variations that don't require getting into a rock-bottom squat.

Another training regime focuses on the clean, leaving out the jerk portion. Solely doing cleans without the jerks over time will develop speed, agility, and power.

So even though the clean and jerk and the snatch are done in competition, you can see there are a wide variety of movements to practice. Practiced on a regular basis, these explosive moves will translate into a more powerful, athletic physique.

CROSSFIT & OLYMPIC WEIGHTLIFTING

Thanks to the fitness phenomenon known as CrossFit, which prominently features the snatch and the clean and jerk in the workout, hundreds of thousands of people now routinely perform Olympic lifts. Like or hate CrossFit, the trend has opened up the world of Olympic weightlifting to ordinary people looking for a way to keep in shape and get strong.

CrossFit trains the Olympic lifts but not in the way that true Olympic weightlifting athletes train. Because Olympic weightlifting is very technical, the trainee must focus on perfecting technique rather than be concerned with how many repetitions are done, how fast the reps are completed, or using a specific weight. True Olympic athletes typically do no more than three to perhaps five reps at most in one set, with several minutes of rest before doing another set. They never train to fatigue as it encourages poor form that, under the heavy loads of the true Olympic athlete, will cause injuries.

Olympic athletes lift hundreds of pounds in both the clean and jerk and the snatch. Doing more than a few reps at a time is a sure road to disaster. It's not uncommon to miss a rep. This means you were unable to complete the rep and failed at some point during the movement. Lifting under fatigue increases the chances for missed lifts, which in turn increases the risk of injury. As with any other sport, Olympic weightlifting requires practice and takes years of training to be good. You train to get better, stronger, faster, and more agile, but all of these attributes worsen under fatigue.

CrossFit takes the approach that their loads are much lighter (typically 95 pounds for women and 135 pounds for men). They supposedly adjust the workout accordingly, but doing 21 clean and jerks with a bar, no matter what the weight, is unwise, especially for beginners. True Olympic lifters, especially at the Olympic level, will move 100 kilograms (220 pounds) or more depending on the lift. Here are a few records in the snatch, the most difficult lift:

MEN'S SNATCH	
WEIGHT CLASS	RECORD
56kg (123.5lbs)	137kg (301.4lbs)
105kg+ (231lbs+)	212kg (466.4lbs)

WOMEN'S SNATCH	
WEIGHT CLASS	RECORD
48kg (105.6lbs)	97kg (213.4lbs)
75kg+ (165lbs+)	187kg (411.4lbs)

Of course, as for you and me, we'll never move that much. The athletes live and breathe Olympic weightlifting and they've been training since they were very young. So how much can you expect to lift? It really depends on your body weight, gender, and experience level, as you can see from the Catalyst Athletics chart below:

	NOVICE MALE 77kg (169.4lbs)	ADVANCED MALE 77kg (169.4lbs)	NOVICE FEMALE 69kg (151.8lb)	ADVANCED FEMALE 69kg (151.8lb)
Snatch	58kg (127.6lbs)	101kg (222.2lbs)	35kg (77lbs)	62kg (136.4lbs)
Clean and Jerk	69kg (151.8lbs)	121kg (266.2lbs)	44kg (96.8lbs)	78kg (171.6lbs)
Back Squat	93kg (204.6lbs)	162kg (356.4lbs)	62kg (136.4lbs)	109kg (239.8lbs)
Front Squat	59kg (129.8lbs)	142kg (312.4lbs)	51kg (112.2lbs)	91kg (200.2lbs)

Source: Catalyst Athletics. To see the full chart, visit www.catalystathletics.com/article/1836/Olympic-Weightlifting-Skill-Levels-Chart

As you can see, there's a big difference in the amount of weight lifted from novice to advanced. To be fair, not all CrossFit gyms follow the same high-rep approach on Olympic lifts. In fact, in the CrossFit community, there are no recognized standards on how the Olympic lifts should be programmed into the workouts. So if you're thinking about joining a CrossFit gym, make sure you personally research the coach. The ideal teaching process is structured and breaks the movements down into easy-to-learn parts. It's also progressive, where you "earn" the right to do more complex movement patterns. Also, the focus should be on technically well-executed lifts rather than on speed/time or completing the reps no matter what.

EQUIPMENT

So you want to Olympic weightlift? Unless you're training at a facility with everything you need, you'll have to buy some gear.

THE BAR. First and foremost, you're going to need an Olympic-sized barbell. The Olympic bar is a little over 7 feet long (men's standard). The ends are 49–50mm in diameter while the shaft is 28–29mm (1.1-inch) thick and weighs 20 kilograms (44 pounds). If you buy a bar in pounds, it'll weight 45 pounds but the other dimensions remain the same. Regardless of the measurement system you use, make sure your plates correspond to the same measurement system as the bar.

If you're serious about Olympic weightlifting, you'll want to invest in a high-quality bar, not the cheap versions often found at sporting-goods stores. Ivanko, Pendlay, Eleiko, and Rogue Fitness all produce top-quality Olympic bars. There are small differences: Some have ball bearings, some use needle bearings, and others use bushings; some are sealed and some aren't. If the bar has hex nuts in the ends or Allen screws in the sleeves, it's *not* suitable for Olympic lifting. You'll also need to consider these following factors.

Flex. True Olympic bars are designed to flex and whip as the bar is pulled up into rack position. The whip adds momentum to the plates, making it a little easier to clean or snatch. As you pull, the bar flexes; as you finish the second portion of the pull, the ends of the bar—and the plates—will continue to move up even though the center of the bar has stopped flexing. A cheap bar will not do that, and under heavy load may even snap.

Don't use a powerlifting bar, either. A powerlifting bar is stiffer with much sharper knurling. The stiff bar won't give you a good whip during the movements and the sharper knurling will cut into your hands.

Rotation. The bar needs to be able to rotate freely while the ends stay fixed. A cheap bar uses inferior components that will prevent the bar from rotating as smoothly as it should, which affects your lifting technique. To create this smooth rotation, bars are made with ball bearings, bushings, or needle bearings. While ball bearings were once the preferred standard, the newer needle bearings are the way to go with your bar. Needle bearings can better withstand the forces applied to them on the lift and when a lifter drops the bar to the ground. Yes, many people drop the barbell after they've gotten it overhead. Over time this will break the bar and you should refrain from doing this unless you miss a lift.

There are three options when it comes to the rotating sleeve: bushings, ball bearings, and needle bearings. Bushings are basically a sleeve that the bar fits through but isn't fixed in place. Bushings don't provide as smooth a rotation compared to needle bearings but can take more punishment. Bars with bushings are okay for the average lifter. Ball bearings provide smoother rotation but are nowhere near as sturdy as a bushing or needle bearings. Some manufacturers use bushing and ball bearings together, which makes them stronger and gives a smoother rotation. However, the best bars use needle bearings, which are longer and provide a more consistent rotation. But bars with needle bearings aren't as durable and are more expensive than bars made with bushings or ball bearings.

My recommendation is to stay away from ball-bearing-only bars. Get a bar with bushings or, if you can afford it, needle bearings.

Knurling. Knurling is the rough part of the bar where the hands go. On an Olympic bar, the knurling is smooth to minimize friction on your hands while the bar is rotating. In comparison, a powerlifting bar has rough knurling to help you keep your grip in the lifts. The placement and length of knurling also differs between the two bar styles.

The International Weightlifting Federation (IWF) requires center knurling on competition bars but you'll find some Olympic bars without the center knurling. It won't really matter for training. If you're doing high-rep cleans in a CrossFit routine, you may prefer a bar without the center knurling, which can rough up your neck a bit. The center knurling is important if you're doing a lot of back squats as it helps keep the bar from slipping from your shirt. If you're lifting shirtless, the center knurl will rough you up.

PLATES. You should always use bumper plates, which are made of solid rubber, usually with a steel ring on the inner edge that slips over the end of the barbell. They're designed to absorb being dropped. The best bumper plates are solid rubber with a fairly wide steel plate. Do not use metal plates! Metal plates will break and ruin the bar if dropped. Mixing bumper and metal plates will also still cause damage to the bar and plates. Even bumper plates have their limits and can break if they're dropped repeatedly.

Bumper plates come in pounds and kilos. For ease of calculating the loads you lift, make sure the units of measurement match the bar you have. That is, if you have a 20-kilogram bar, your plates should also be in kilos. Conversely, a 45-pound bar should be used with plates in pounds.

MAINTAIN YOUR BAR

You should keep the exterior of the bar and knurling clean. Chalk builds up in the knurling, reducing its effectiveness. In addition, old sweat will cause the bar to rust. To clean the bar, use a nylon brush to scrub off the chalk and dirt. When the bar is clean, use 3-in-1 oil on the bar and let it sit for an hour or so then wipe it off with a clean cloth.

You'll also periodically need to oil the bearings so they continue to rotate freely. Each manufacturer will have its own way of oiling the bearings/bushings. It may require you to take the bar apart to clean the area where the bearings contact the bar. Do not use WD-40 to lube the bar. Typically the bearings will be lubricated with grease, a non-detergent oil, or 3-in-1 oil.

PRICING BARS & BUMPERS

Top-quality bumpers and bars will run you thousands of dollars, but you can get a good quality bar for $200-$300 and a complete set of decent plates for about the same amount. Check around on Craigslist, the usual online shops, or Google "Olympic bars" and "Olympic bumper plates" for the best deals.

COLLARS. Collars keep the plates from falling off the bar. Do *not* lift without collars—if you lose control of the bar and it tips to one side, the plates will fall off and could seriously injure you. Look for a good-quality pair of collars. When you're starting off with lighter weights, using the spring variety might suffice (they'll run you about $10 pair). As you progress to working heavy, you'll need a heavy-duty set, which costs about $40. Don't skimp on this vital part of your Olympic weightlifting set.

PLATFORM. You shouldn't lift on bare concrete or a wood floor. Concrete will tear up the plates and bar and you'll put holes in the wood floor. Ideally you'll want an Olympic lifting platform made of plywood with a veneer, and rubber flooring in the middle portion. The prices range from $300 up to well over $1200.

JERK BLOCKS. Jerk blocks or boxes elevate the bar from the ground, which allows you to work on specific parts of the clean and the snatch. You can buy a variety of boxes made specifically for Olympic weightlifting work or make your own (Google "build jerk blocks" for directions on how to make your own for around $200).

Blocks are useful tools for refining your form or focusing on weaker portions of your pull. For example, if you don't do well pulling from the floor because you lack hip mobility, the blocks allow you to work within your range of motion without risking bad back position or faulty technique. You should, of course, be working to improve that hip mobility.

Use taller blocks to focus on jerks without the clean portion. You can even use the boxes as you would a squat rack so, if you're squatting, the boxes can be used to check depth or (if you lose it) to catch the bar.

SHOES. If you're really serious about the sport, invest in good-quality Olympic weightlifting shoes, which are very firm with an elevated heel that helps you get into that rock-bottom squat when doing full Olympic cleans or snatches. The elevated heel overcomes lack of ankle dorsiflexion, which will prevent you from getting deep into a squat, cause your torso to fall too far forward, or cause your knees to go too far forward or inward (valgus). If you choose to not use Olympic weightlifting shoes, get a pair of Chuck Taylor Converse or other solid-sole shoes. Don't use cross-trainers or running shoes—they don't provide the needed support in the ankle and arches. In addition, they're designed to absorb energy, which will take power away from your lifts.

There's some physiology at work here in the feedback mechanisms between your feet, legs, and brain that the squishy shoes mess up. Basically, there are sensors in your feet that provide feedback to your brain. Being barefoot or in firm shoes keeps that feedback intact. Using soft, energy-absorbing shoes limits the feedback, thereby limiting information to the brain, which should be telling the legs to produce force in response to the pressure in the feet.

BELTS & STRAPS. Beginner- to intermediate-level weightlifters should avoid using the belt until they're working with heavy weights daily. Once you're regularly using heavy weights, invest in a belt.

Some lifters also use lifting straps that loop around the bar and each hand. The straps take the grip out of the equation as well, eliminating the problem many have of tight wrists and forearms in the rack position. However, I don't necessarily recommend this on a long-term basis as I think you need to work on strengthening your grip to improve your wrist and forearm mobility.

CHALK. Lifting chalk, made from magnesium carbonate, improves your grip. You can get a six-block box for around $15. A box should last a while (at my gym we go through a full box every six months or so). You can also get chalk in a bag, designed for climbers so they can attach it to their belt or climbing harness for easy access. The chalk bag cuts down on the mess. If you use blocks, you'll want to keep them in a bucket or box. Don't use chalk made for playing pool. Made with talcum, pool chalk has the opposite effect—it makes your grip slippery.

RECORDING DEVICE. It's always a good idea to record your sets, especially if you don't have a coach watching and fixing your technique. Record your lifts and then review the footage to see where your form may be breaking down or what needs to be tweaked. If you have a long-distance coach (e.g., one you're working with over Skype), you'll be able to send the clip to your coach for evaluation. If you don't have a video camera, an iPad, tablet, or smartphone will work, too.

PLYO BOXES. A set of three plyo boxes (18-inch, 20-inch, and 24-inch heights) is useful for doing box jumps, a plyometric exercise that improves your explosiveness. If you have flat jerk boxes, the taller versions can be used as well.

ROLLERS, BALLS, STICKS, & BANDS. Your muscles and associated tissue get stiff whether you exercise or not. If you've ever had a massage and the therapist found a place that hurt a lot to the touch, you've experienced a trigger point. Or perhaps you get headaches for no reason; these can be caused by trigger points or a mechanism known as referred pain. A good massage therapist can help get rid of these tight spots, but the next best thing is what's known as self-myofascial release (SMFR). *Myo* means "muscles" and *fascial* refers to the "fascia," tissue that covers and connects all the muscles throughout the body.

Foam rollers and *lacrosse balls* are ideal at-home solutions. Rolling them across your back, legs, and hips, looking for tender areas, will help release the tissue. You can pick up foam roller online or in most sporting-goods stores; the denser the better. If you find that lacrosse balls are too hard at first, use a firm tennis ball.

You can also buy a *stick massager* that looks like a rolling pin. Two popular brands are The Stick and the Tiger Tail. This rigid roller performs the same function as the foam roller but can reach areas that the foam roller or ball doesn't work well on, such as the calves. It's readily available online at Amazon.com or PerformBetter.com.

The *resistance band* is for stretching and available online and in sporting-goods stores. Make sure to get one with about 30 pounds of resistance. Don't use rehab bands (what you get if you go through physical therapy, or what you'll find in most department and sporting-goods stores)—they're too light for our purposes and will break. We need to create resistance heavy enough to build reactive strength in the body, not just rehab an injury.

SAFETY

If you're healthy, you should be able to do the Olympic lifts and most of the variations with little trouble. However, you should also make sure you have no prior injuries or shoulder mobility problems. Jerks and snatches involve bringing weight overhead, which necessitates strong shoulders. The clean by itself is a great exercise to develop explosive power and speed, and bad shoulders shouldn't present a problem in most cases.

As with any exercise program, see your doctor to make sure doing the exercises in this book will not cause you problems. If your physician doesn't know about Olympic weightlifting, find a good physical therapist and have an evaluation done prior to starting any Olympic lifts.

Once you consult with your doctor and/or physical therapist, here are some guidelines to follow when doing Olympic weightlifting.

BEFORE YOU LIFT

CLEAR THE LIFTING AREA. There should be nothing on the platform except you and the bar—make sure the lifting area is free of obstructions such as extra bars, plates, or collars. If you miss a lift, any extra equipment can make it harder to safely escape the falling bar. All it takes is one misstep—or trip—to seriously injure yourself.

SAFETY CHECKLIST

Whether you're a long-time lifter or first timer, you should always go through these safety tips.

- Clear the lifting area.
- Check bar for damage.
- Check weight and dimensions of plates on both sides of the bar.
- Check the plates for cracks.
- Check the collars for damage; they also should be a matching pair.
- Check that the collars are properly securing the plates.
- Check the lifting boxes for damage and weight limit (they must be able to hold the weight that you're lifting).
- Check the squat rack for any abnormal wear and tear.

Case in point: One of the best CrossFitters in the country overdid it at a CrossFit competition. He missed the lift and fell, landing against a stack of plates with his bar falling right onto him. He broke his spine and was paralyzed from the waist down. So give yourself ample room to escape a lift if needed.

CHECK YOUR EQUIPMENT. First off, check your bar for damage and, if applicable, make sure the sleeves are screwed in tight. On some less-expensive models, the sleeves are held on by a screw, or screws. The screws should be securely fastened.

You'll also need to make sure you have the same size, weight, and number of plates on each side (i.e., if you have two 25-pound weights on the left side, you need two 25-pound weights on the right side rather than one 50-pound plate). If the number of plates is uneven, this tends to make the bar lean to the side with more plates due to the offset center of gravity, increasing the risk of dropping the bar. If your bar is supported on a squat rack and you have to change the bumper plates, load and unload one plate at a time, alternating sides. If you take all the plates off one side first, the bar will become unbalanced and fall off the hooks.

Also check for cracks in the plates. If a plate is cracked and you drop the bar, the defective plate may damage the floor/platform and the bar. A cracked plate could possibly come apart while you're lifting it, causing serious injury. Examine the collars to ensure that they're undamaged and are properly securing the plates. Use collars rated for Olympic weightlifting and always use the same type on either side of the bar. Don't use a spring collar on one side and a clamp collar on the other—it's not smart to mix safety equipment.

Any boxes used should be undamaged and strong enough to hold the weight you're lifting. Review squat racks (J-hooks and other components) for abnormal wear and tear.

ESCAPING A MISSED LIFT

If you miss a hang clean, simply push the bar forward and move backward. Missing a full clean is trickier. However, even missing at rock bottom you can get away by pushing the bar forward and jumping backward.

Getting out from under a snatch can be a little more difficult but, basically, you need to move in the opposite direction of the bar. So if the snatch is missed going overhead (the most common miss), the bar will be heading behind you. Release the bar (which will continue on its backward trajectory) while simultaneously moving yourself forward quickly.

If you miss the snatch or otherwise lose control of it while at the bottom of a squat and the bar is overhead, you'll have to quickly determine which way the bar wants to fall, let it go, and move in the opposite direction as quickly as possible.

NUTRITION

Eating right is an important part of any fitness program, but with so many next-great-diets out there with conflicting information, what's right? Paleo this, gluten-free that. No fat, no carbs, no animals. South Beach, Atkins, Ornish. Arrgghh, it makes my head hurt and makes me want to scream!

I'm going to tell you the secret to being healthy, losing fat (if you need to) or gaining muscle (if you want). Normally you'd have to pay thousands for this top-secret information (really, I saw it on Facebook so it must be true) but I'm giving it to you for the price of this book.

Wait for it. Are you ready? Don't eat processed foods. Bam. Top-secret stuff there.

Seriously, though, eliminating processed foods will kickstart fat loss and help increase muscle by getting you to eat real foods with an emphasis on increasing your lean protein intake to about 35 percent of your daily calories.

A good rule of thumb: If it comes in a box or a bag, it's probably processed. There are exceptions, such as a bag of fresh-frozen vegetables or a box of steel-cut oats. But by and large, if it's in a box or bag, it's processed.

Processing foods is typically done to improve shelf life or change the flavor of something. It's done by adding chemicals, including coloring and preservatives—all of which can be potentially harmful to your health. Manufacturers also like to sneak in fats, salt, and sugar, the three things your brain craves and you can become addicted to. This makes it much more likely you'll eat more and continue to buy the "food."

PROTEIN. Your body needs protein as much as it needs fats. Technically, you can survive without carbs, but you can't live without protein. In addition to building muscles, protein is essential for healthy bones, hair, nails, and skin—basically the raw fuel for virtually every cell in your body. Animal proteins contain many essential nutrients without which your body will start to break down. For example, many vegans need B12 shots because their protein sources don't naturally have it.

Other essential nutrients that can only be obtained from animal protein sources include branched chain amino acids (BCAAs), which help promote muscle building and the production of creatine, a compound used as a source of fuel in short, intense bursts of activity (like a 100-meter sprint).

One of the biggest myths about protein is that too much of it will ruin your kidneys—no study has ever proven that to be true. However, if you have kidney issues, you may need to reduce your protein intake—consult with your doctor. Otherwise getting 30–35 percent of your daily calories from protein should not be a problem.

There's a lot of disagreement about how much protein a person needs. The U.S. Recommended Daily Allowance (RDA) for men is a measly 54 grams of protein. However, current research says that you need .75–1 gram of protein for every pound of lean muscle mass you have. If you're a 175-pound male with 25 percent body fat who's training hard, you'd actually need at least 130 grams of protein, almost 80 grams more than the RDA, especially if your goal is to pack on muscle.

Even if you're trying to lose fat, it's important to keep your protein intake consistent with your calculated protein needs—you'll lose body fat whether you fill the remaining daily caloric requirements with more carbs and less fats *or* less fats and more carbs. Of course, the total daily calorie allotment must be the same regardless of the carb/fat ratio. For example, if you require 2000 calories a day and you're getting 700 calories from protein, whether you get 800 calories from carbs and 500 from fat or the other way around, the effects will be the same in the long run.

There are hundreds of studies showing the importance of protein in the diet, including research that points to accelerated fat loss by adding more lean protein and cutting carbs (but not below 20 percent or so). In essence, it seems that it doesn't really matter if you're on a low-fat or a low-carb plan—protein is the key.

RULES FOR HEALTHY EATING

Here are a few simple guidelines for maintaining a proper diet.

1. Eat lean protein with every meal.

2. Eat vegetables with every meal.

3. If you're trying to lose fat, stay away from starchy carbs except after a workout.

4. Avoid sugary foods and drinks.

5. Drink water—at least half your body weight in ounces—every day.

6. Avoid *all* soft drinks.

7. Avoid alcohol.

8. Watch your portion sizes.

9. If you're fairly knowledgeable about nutrition, are doing well with your diet, and still want to get leaner, you may need to count calories plus track your macronutrients.

There's no way you can be 100 percent compliant for long, so shoot for 90 percent adherence to these rules. This means it's okay to eat pizza on a Saturday night as long as you get right back on track the next day.

Look at it this way: If you eat 4 meals per day (counting snacks), that's 28 meals per week. That means you can keep to clean-eating 25 meals with 3 cheat meals per week and still do fine.

SOFT DRINKS & ALCOHOL

Don't drink soft drinks. Besides the high sugar content, the added chemicals can wreck havoc on your body. I'm sure you've seen the videos where Coke is used to clean pennies and toilets—that's the phosphoric acid eating away at the dirt. Yes, it can eat your insides as well if you consume a lot of sodas every day.

While sugar in soft drinks is bad for you, artificial sweeteners are even worse. They trick the brain into thinking it's getting sugar and, until the brain and body get actual sugar, you'll continue to eat or drink. In fact, current studies are showing causation between consumption of artificial sweeteners and obesity.

You don't need to eliminate alcohol in your diet—just drink sensibly. Imbibe on an empty stomach (yes, you read that right) and make sure you don't have more than two drinks. To prevent fat gain, alcohol should be consumed on an empty stomach, or eat only lean protein before drinking. The science is that alcohol is a toxin and the body shuts down all fat and carb burning until the alcohol is removed from the system. So instead of being burned off, carbs and fats immediately get shoved into storage. Also avoid mixed drinks like margaritas—there's a lot of added sugar. If hard liquor is your preference, order it straight up, on the rocks, or cut with water.

VEGETABLES. Eat vegetables with every meal—they're loaded with vitamins and minerals. Most people don't eat anywhere nearly enough veggies as they should and require supplements to get adequate levels of some nutrients.

In addition, vegetables are dense and fibrous and you can eat a lot of them before getting full. While starchy carbs fill you up faster, you get hungry faster, too, which promotes overeating.

Go for a rainbow of vegetables: greens such as spinach, kale, broccoli, and green beans; red veggies such as peppers and beets; orange/yellow options like carrots, butternut squash, and sweet corn; blue/purple vegetables like eggplant and endive. Remember to be smart about preparing your vegetables, too. A little butter (never, ever use margarine!) and salt is okay, but don't slather your veggies with them, either.

SIMPLE CARBOHYDRATES & SUGARY FOODS. Starchy and sugary foods, or simple carbohydrates, keep you satiated for a shorter period of time compared to consuming protein and fats. Thus, you end up hungry sooner and eat more, contributing to overeating.

Your body breaks down sugary or starchy foods into glucose, storing what it needs to maintain stable blood sugar levels and for energy. When the stores are full, glucose is transported to other cells for use. Once the glucose is stored for energy or absorbed in the cells, any remaining glucose is stored as fat.

This is one reason why, if you do eat starchy carbs, you should do so within an hour *after* a good workout. You want to replenish the glucose and glycogen stores so your overall blood sugar stays at normal levels.

I don't recommend a pre-workout drink or meal that's sugary or starchy. The reason? Glucose stored for energy will be used before glucose stored as fat, so if you eat foods that produce an abundance of glucose, your body will use the stored glucose before burning fat.

However, if you eat sensibly and only consume starchy carbs or sweet fruit after a workout, you'll be just fine. Yes, fruit contains sugar in the form of fructose, but it also contains a plethora of important vitamins necessary for proper health. Just don't go overboard.

WATER. Most people don't drink enough water. The easiest way to tell if you're properly hydrated is by checking the color of your urine. If it's pale yellow to clear, you're probably getting enough water. If it's yellow or darker, you need more water. (If it's dark brown, you need to go to the hospital ASAP!)

The rule of thumb is to drink half your body weight in ounces of water. Some people will count unsweetened tea with this, but not coffee. Your body is 70 percent water so if you're dehydrated, your body will start to shut down.

Don't overdo your water intake, though. Too much water and not enough salt will trigger hyponatremia, a state where the sodium levels in your body are too low. Some symptoms include dizziness, vomiting, headaches, nausea, short-term memory loss, lethargy, and fatigue. If you sweat a lot during exercise, *do* drink water but perhaps supplement your drink with some salt to help keep the water/salt ratio in the proper range.

OLYMPIC WEIGHTLIFTING BASICS

While the following are basic positions, they're very important. Failure to master them means a failure to reach your full potential in the Olympic lifts. The foot positions will be what feels natural to you, perhaps with a little tweaking. The rack position requires flexible wrists, elbows, and shoulders—if you're tight in those areas, a good rack position will be tough to hit, making your cleans less efficient.

The hang position is important both as a starting point for the hang versions of the clean and snatch and as a transition point when doing both lifts from the floor. If you don't understand the hang position and how it differs between cleans and snatches, you'll have problems generating force and being able to lift heavier weights.

HANG POSITION. Midway through the first pull, the bar is a little above knee level, the hips are not yet fully extended, and the torso is still inclined. This is the hang position for the clean and snatch, which is used a lot for training the movement segments as well as for those who struggle with the first pull. This term is also used for a point in time for the clean or snatch from the floor. The clean hang position (page 83) uses a hook grip. There's also a snatch version (page 118) that uses a wide hook grip, which makes the position a little deeper.

RACK POSITION. You're in rack position when the bar is across the fronts of your shoulders, resting on the tips of your fingers, and lightly touching your throat. The upper arms should be parallel to the floor. See the rack position directions (page 83) in the Clean chapter for directions on how to get into the position.

KETTLEBELL RACK POSITION. In the kettlebell rack position, the bell rests against the back of your forearm, with your elbow tight to your side and into your ribs, and your palm angled toward your body. The bell's handle sits on the bone on the heel of your hand, below your pinky and across to the webbing of your thumb/forefinger. The handle of the bell should be at or slightly below your clavicle (collarbone).

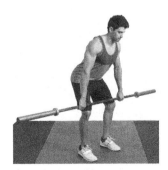
Clean hang position

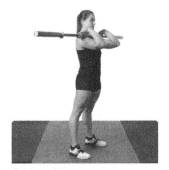
Rack position

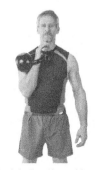
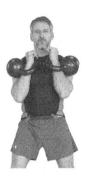
Kettlebell rack position

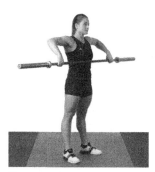

Scarecrow

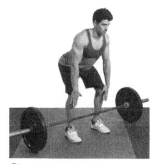

Short-stop position

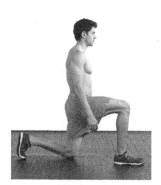

Half-kneeling position

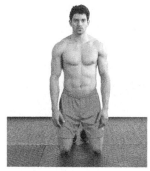

Tall-kneeling position

SCARECROW POSITION. Scarecrow position is a point in time during the clean and the snatch where the bar has traveled up to about chest level with the elbows as high as they can go before the turnover into rack position (the clean) or getting the bar overhead (the snatch). The scarecrow position allows us to isolate a very short, fast part of cleans and snatches.

SHORT-STOP POSITION. This position is named for its resemblance to the stance of a baseball player at short stop. Stand tall with your feet shoulder-width apart, hands on your thighs. Push your hips back and let the knees bend slightly. The hands slide down the thighs to rest on the knees. Your chest is out and spine is neutral.

STARTING FOOT POSITION. This is called the *pulling stance* for both the clean and the snatch: feet hip-width apart, not any wider, and turned out slightly. In the jerk, the starting position is referred to as the *drive stance*.

ENDING FOOT POSITION. This varies depending on the lift and whether you're doing a full version or the power version. In the clean, the ending foot position is called a *squat stance*; in the snatch it's the *catch stance*. For the jerk, you'll either end in a *parallel stance* (feet slightly out to the side) or *split stance* (one foot in front and the other in back).

HALF-KNEELING POSITION. This stance is also known as the 90/90 position. To get into the half-kneeling position from standing, get on one knee.

- The foot, knee, and hip of the lead leg should be aligned. You can check by using a stick or your forearm to make sure the knee and foot are directly in front of the hip and the hips are straight ahead.

- The shin of the lead leg should be vertical.

- The rear knee should be directly under the rear hip; the rear thigh should be vertical from the front and from the side.

- You should be on the ball of the rear foot and it should be directly behind the knee, which should be in line with the hips.

- Picture headlights on your hip bones and shoulders. The headlights should point straight ahead.

TALL-KNEELING POSITION. From standing, get on both knees.

- Your knees should be positioned under the hips but not together.

- Your thighs should be vertical from the front and sides.

ARE YOU READY TO OLYMPIC LIFT?

You may be mentally ready to start Olympic lifting but are you physically prepared? In this section we cover some easy self-assessments to make sure you're clear for training the Olympic lifts. If you do find problems or weaknesses, we'll show you how to improve those areas. Be safe, not sorry. Since the self-assessments can only go so far in uncovering problems, before you begin, get checked out by a good doctor or physical therapist.

These assessments are based on the Functional Movement Screen (FMS), a system developed by Gray Cook and Lee Burton. The FMS has been used on thousands of professional athletes to determine their risks for injury, as well as give them the tools to get moving well. The screens intentionally place you in extreme positions to see how you handle them or compensate.

The screens are the Overhead Squat (OHS), Hurdle Step (HS), Inline Lunge (ILL), Shoulder Mobility (SM), Active Straight-Leg Raise (ASLR), Trunk Stability Push-Up (TSPU), and Rotational Stability (RS). The correctives or fixes are done from the most primitive (ASLR and SM) to the transitional patterns (TSPU and RS), then up to the HS, ILL, and OHS.

Typically, if there's a problem with one of the "Big Three" (HS, ILL, OHS), the fix lies in one of the more basic "little four" (SM, ASLR, TSPU, RS). What this means is that if you have a tough time with the overhead squat, which is part of the snatch, you need to look at the lower-level movement patterns and clear them. Those fixes should translate into a better overhead squat.

I've modified the screens to make it easy to assess yourself. If you want to do the full screen, you'll need to find a certified FMS professional (functionalmovement.com/experts).

Each assessment is followed by suggested exercise fixes that will clean up your restricted or weak movement patterns. The correctives covered have been proven to work on most people most of the time. Some of these fixes will clear up a movement problem quickly, but other issues may take longer. Do the exercise fixes every day, not just training days. The more often you do them, the faster you'll get cleared to do Olympic lifts.

Pick two or three fixes for each screen you have problems with. If you try to do each one, you'll spend all day doing nothing but correctives. If you have multiple areas that need work, remember to start with and focus on the ASLR and SM. Pick one or two fixes for each one and don't spend more than 5 minutes working them.

Again, these screens show poor movement patterns caused by weakness or imbalance. If you have any pain, see your doctor or physical therapist before embarking on a lifting program.

SQUAT & SHOULDER MOBILITY ASSESSMENT

If you don't have shoulder mobility, you won't be able to safely execute the jerk portion of the clean and jerk. The following assessments go from simple to advanced and are designed to progressively pinpoint the areas that need strengthening.

In this functional movement screen, we look at the entire overhead squat pattern, but it has been my experience that most people can't do it so I like to look at some smaller parts of it first.

SCORING THE SCREENS

For this book you'll score yourself on a pass/fail basis; either you can do the movement or you can't. If you fail on more than 2 of these screens, you aren't physically ready to do the Olympic lifts. I highly encourage you to seek out a qualified FMS trainer who can help you rebuild your foundational movements. FMS pros will also do a clearing test on the SM, TSPU, and RS patterns to look for pain that might not have occurred in the screen.

For example, as part of the SM screen we check for shoulder impingement because pain means there's an underlying issue that a doctor needs to check out, as most FMS pros aren't physical therapists or doctors. It's a little challenging to self-score as we want to think we're better than we are. I highly recommend recording your screen so you can go back and see it rather than trying to feel it out.

SA 1: Overhead Wall Touch

If you know you don't have any shoulder problems you can move on to SA 2.

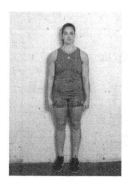 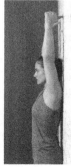

1. Stand with your back to the wall with your head, upper back, and tailbone touching the wall.   **2.** With your hands in fists, palms facing each other, and thumbs extended, raise both arms straight up overhead. Try to touch the wall with your thumbs.

SCORING **Pass:** You can touch the wall with your thumbs without arching your back. Do SA 2 or SA 3. **Fail:** You couldn't touch the wall with your thumbs or any part of your back, or any part of your back lost contact with the wall. Do SA 4.

SA 2: Overhead Squat

This is the main screen.

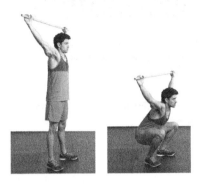

1. Stand with your feet shoulder-width apart. With a wide overhand grip, press a broomstick or 5-foot PVC pipe overhead and keep it there.   **2.** With your arms overhead and elbows locked out, squat down slowly and deliberately. At the same time drive your knees out so they remain pointed in the same direction as your toes. Go as deep as you can.

SCORING Pass: Arms are overhead, torso is upright, shins are parallel to torso—you're good to go for overhead work, including overhead squats, full snatches, and jerks. Move on to the Hurdle Step Assessment (page 32). **Fail:** Arms are in front of body, torso is folded over, hips are not level with or below the knees, heels are off the ground. Do SA 3.

SA 3: Overhead Squat with Elevated Heel

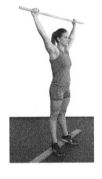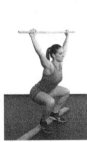

1. Stand with your feet shoulder-width apart and your heels elevated on a 2x4 or 2x6 board. With a wide overhand grip, hold a broomstick or 5-foot-long PVC pipe overhead.   **2.** Squat down slowly and deliberately. At the same time drive your knees out so they remain pointed in the same direction as your toes. Go as deep as you can.

SCORING Pass: Arms are overhead, torso and shins are parallel to each other, hips are level with or below the knees. Work on your ankle flexibility. **Fail:** Arms are in front on body, torso and shins are not parallel, body is folded over, hips are above the knees. Work on core strength, shoulder mobility and strength, hip mobility and strength, and ankle mobility.

If you struggled with SA 3, do SA 4. Otherwise move on to the Hurdle Step Assessment (page 32).

If you failed any of the above screens, you shouldn't do snatches or jerks. You can still do power cleans since you don't have to get into a full squat.

SA 4: Bodyweight Squat

I use this as a screen when someone tells me he's having trouble with his arms overhead. This way I can still screen the basic squat pattern without worrying about causing harm. If you don't have shoulder problems then you don't need to do this.

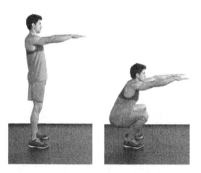

1. Stand with your feet slightly wider than shoulder width and turned out a little. Extend your arms in front of you, parallel to the floor. **2.** Squat down slowly and deliberately. At the same time drive your knees out so they remain pointed in the same direction as your toes. Go as deep as you can.

SCORING Pass: Feet are flat on floor, hips are level with or below knees, torso and shins parallel to each other, there's no shifting of the hips to one side, no knee collapse. You can squat but should not do full snatches. **Fail:** Torso collapses, heels come off the floor, knees cave in, shifting to one side at any time. Work on hip mobility and strength, core strength, and ankle mobility.

FIXES If you had trouble with SA 1 (you couldn't touch the wall or your back arched), you need to get your shoulder blades and upper back moving. If you had no problems with SA 1, you don't need to do any of these.

FIX 1: Quad Extension Rotation (page 170)

FIX 2: Forearm Wall Slide (page 170)

FIX 3: Back-to-Wall Arm Slide (page 170)

FIX 4: Band-Assisted Pec Stretch (page 171)

FIX 5: Spiderman with Rotation (page 171)

FIX 6: Halo (page 171)

FIX 7: Shoulder Dislocate (page 172)

FIX 8: Side-Lying Windmill (page 172)

FIX 9: Bretzel (page 173)

FIX 10: Lat Stretch with Band (page 173)

FIX 11: Arm Bar (page 173)

Problems with SA 2 and SA 3 indicate that your ankles are restricted. Pick two or three of these if you failed the screen.

FIX 1: Standing Knee-to-Wall Ankle Mobility (page 174)

FIX 2: Toe Pull 1 (page 174) or Toe Pull 2 (page 174)

FIX 3: Calf Stretch (page 175)

FIX 4: Lower Legs Roller Release (page 175)

Problems doing SA 4 probably mean you have tight hips. Pick one or two of these fixes.

FIX 1: Hip Rock Back (page 175)

FIX 2: Leg-Abducted Rock Back (page 176)

FIX 3: Face-the-Wall Squat (page 176)

FIX 4: Bootstrapper (page 154)

You don't need to do fixes for all four sections. Pick a few from the SA that gave you the most trouble.

Hurdle Step Assessment

This movement is pertinent to jerks as well as any jumping movement, especially box jumps or running. This assessment looks at your hip mobility and core stability.

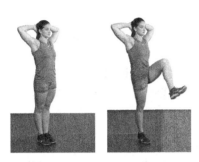

1. Stand with your hands behind your head. **2.** Lift one knee up as high as you can. **3.** Lower it to the floor. Repeat once more then twice on the other leg.

This screen checks both sides of the body. You might pass on one side and fail on the other. That's an asymmetry that will need to be cleared up.

When doing the unilateral fixes, focus on the weaker side.

SCORING **Pass:** Thigh is above parallel, there's no movement anywhere except the knee coming up. **Fail:** Couldn't get thigh above parallel or you bent forward to get the knee higher than parallel; you lost your balance.

Remember to score both sides.

FIXES Being able to raise your knee higher than your shin indicates good hip mobility and psoas activation (the psoas runs from the spine through the pelvis and to the inside of the femur) as well as core strength and balance. Without these attributes, you'll have problems with box jumps, squats, and running.

FIX 1: Half-Kneeling Hip Flexor Stretch (page 180)

FIX 2: Marching in Place (page 164)

Lunge Assessment

Since the jerk is a dynamic split squat, you need to be able to do lunges and split squats correctly. If you have problems with this assessment, split jerks will cause you problems. Running with a "fail" or being asymmetrical on this screen tends to cause problems in the hips and knees. This assessment checks to see how your hips are moving and whether you're tight in your hip flexors. *Note for FMS pros:* Normally I use the FMS kit but most people won't have access to it and doing it this way works well as a substitute.

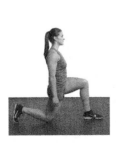
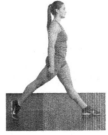

1. Place one knee on the ground. The forward knee is bent 90 degrees with the shin vertical. The middle toe and the center of the knee are aligned with each other. Your hips and torso should point straight forward. The trailing leg should be at a 90-degree angle at the hip. The outside and front of your thigh should be vertical. The ball of your rear foot—not the top of the foot—should be in contact with the floor. Remember this position; it's called the 90/90 or half-kneeling position. **2.** Stand up.

3. Lower your back knee to the floor.   **4.** Repeat once more then switch legs and do the screen twice on the other leg.

Repeat twice on each side.

SCORING Pass: You were able to stand up and stay tall, maintain balance, not move your feet, and keep your torso vertical. **Fail:** You couldn't stand up, you had to use your hands, your lost your balance, your torso pitched forward, or you lost hip alignment.

Remember to score both sides.

FIXES Fix 1 loosens up your hip flexors while Fix 2 strengthens the glutes and core.

FIX 1: Half-Kneeling Hip Flexor Stretch (page 180)

FIX 2: One-Leg Glute Bridge (page 177)

Shoulder Mobility Assessment 2

The Overhead Squat Assessment (page 30) already shows shoulder mobility but only in one area. The shoulders have a wide range of motion and you'll need to check them in different positions. *Note for FMS pros:* This is another modification of the actual screen but a person can't tell how close together his hands are and measuring the gap is impossible.

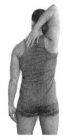 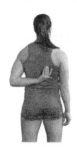

SCRATCH TEST. Try to scratch the top of your right shoulder blade with your left hand moving behind your head. Now try to scratch the lower part of your right shoulder blade with your left hand reaching behind your back. Repeat on the right and note the results.

The true Shoulder Mobility screen is to try and bring your fists as close together as possible behind your back but without forcing it. This version is a modification but will still show the same problems.

SCORING Pass: You were able to scratch the top of the opposite shoulder blade and the bottom of the opposite shoulder blade without arching your back or moving your head. **Fail:** You were unable to scratch either the top or bottom of the opposite shoulder blade, or you had to arch your back to move your head excessively to reach.

Remember to score both sides.

IMPINGEMENT TEST 1. Place your left hand on your right shoulder.   **2.** Raise your left elbow up and down a few times, keeping your hand on your shoulder.

Was there pain?

Repeat the clearance test on the right shoulder. If there's pain in either shoulder, you most likely have an impingement and need to see a doctor. You shouldn't do any overhead exercises until it's cleared up.

FIXES The fixes we looked at previously all had to do with raising the arms overhead, getting mobility in the thoracic spine, and learning to stabilize the shoulder complex. The following movements are designed to work the shoulders and upper back in different planes of movement.

If you had pain on the impingement test, don't do these!

All of the fixes in SA 1 (page 31) apply here.

Active Straight-Leg Raise (ASLR) Assessment

This screen checks to see how well you can control your pelvis and whether your hips can move independently of one another and the rest of your body.

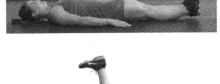

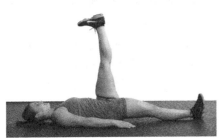

1. Lie flat on your back on the floor with your legs straight and in line with your hips. Pull your toes back toward your shins. **2.** Slowly raise one leg up with control until your knee bends or your leg is vertical. **3.** Lower the leg and repeat on the same side. Switch sides and repeat twice.

SCORING **Pass:** You were able to raise the leg to vertical with no knee bend and no other movement anywhere else, especially in the other leg. **Fail:** Your knee bent before the leg was more than 45 degrees elevated or your other leg moved (including foot turnout).

Remember, if you're asymmetrical, focus on the unilateral fixes on the weak side. Remember to score both sides.

If you're asymmetrical or failed this screen, you shouldn't do any deadlifts, Olympic lifts, kettlebells swings, or other movements involving hip extension.

FIXES If you were asymmetrical, you need to balance yourself out by working the hips/glutes on the weaker side. For example, with the One-Leg Glute Bridge, you should only work the weak-side hip by placing that foot on the floor and lifting the hip.

FIX 1: Glute Bridge, both feet on the floor (page 179); as you get stronger, add the Weighted Glute Bridge (page 179).

FIX 2: Leg Lowering 1 (page 176)

FIX 3: One-Leg Glute Bridge (page 177)

FIX 4: Leg Lowering 2 (page 177)

FIX 5: Bent-Knee Dead Bug (page 178); as you get stronger, progress to Straight-Leg Dead Bug (page 178)

FIX 6: Weighted Glute Bridge (page 179) or Barbell Hip Thruster (page 179)

Trunk Stability Push-Up (TSPU)

The ability to do a push-up while maintaining a neutral stable spine shows good core stability. Lack of static core will affect dynamic core control, especially in deadlifts and squats. Even if you have a great plank, being able to maintain the neutral spine while moving under load may still be difficult.

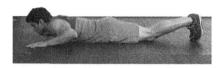

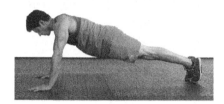

1. Lie facedown with your legs straight. Place your hands so that your thumbs are in line with your forehead (men) or your chin (women). Your elbows should be bent 90 degrees and pointed out to the sides.   **2.** Perform a push-up then lower yourself so that you're lying on the floor.

SCORING Pass: Your body moved in perfect unison on the way up. **Fail:** Your torso came up before your lower body.

PAIN CLEARANCE TEST 1. With your hands in normal push-up position, raise your upper body off the floor by straightening your elbows and keeping your hips down.

Was there any pain in your lower back or shoulders? If so, see your doctor.

FIXES If you had trouble with this assessment, you need to build upper-body strength and core stability. Proper form for almost all exercises (including squats, deadlifts) requires the body to have a neutral spine.

FIX 1: Forearm Plank (page 181) with a 2-minute time goal without deviation

FIX 2: High Plank (page 182) with a 2-minute time goal without losing position

When doing push-ups during your workout, elevate your hands on a box or step high enough to allow you to successfully perform a proper push-up.

Rotary Stability

The Rotary Stability screen looks at your ability to maintain neutral spine while on your hands and knees (Quadruped Position). Your ability to control your torso on one hand and knee (think crawling) and your ability to flex your spine while staying stable are all signs of core stability and rotational control.

The screen looks like a bird dog but is a little different.

The RS screen involves the obliques, the part of your abs that make up your sides. The primary job of the obliques is to prevent torso rotation and create power when trunk rotation is necessary (like when playing tennis or golf). However, when doing one-limb exercises such as one-legged deadlifts, rows, or even standard squats and deadlifts, you want to avoid torso rotation.

You also want to avoid torso rotation in Olympic weightlifting. Weak obliques, especially unbalanced ones, can cause the torso to twist when under load. If one side is stronger than the other, you'll tend to rotate toward the stronger side, causing rotation in the spine that can lead to injury.

In the FMS, the RS is first done with the arm and the same-side leg but in all the people I've screened, no one has been able to do it so these days I skip it..

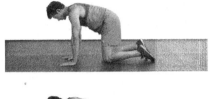
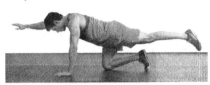
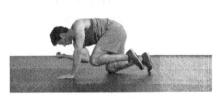

1. Start with your hands under your shoulders (arms vertical and in line with your shoulders) and both knees on the floor, under your hips. The balls of your feet are on the floor. Your fingers should be touching each other, not spread apart.   **2.** Raise one arm directly in front of you and the opposite leg directly behind you. Your hips and shoulders should remain parallel to the floor. Remember: You're going across the body, right foot and left hand and vice versa. The arm and the leg should not be higher than your torso, but they don't have to be parallel to the floor, either.   **3.** Hold the position briefly then try to touch your elbow and knee together under your stomach.   **4.** Extend your arm and leg back out then put them back on the floor to return to start position. Do one more rep on this side then switch sides and repeat. As you switch sides, note any shifting of the body.

SCORING Pass: You were able to extend the arm and opposite leg without any shifting of your body and you were able to bring the knee and elbow together in the centerline without shifting or losing balance. **Fail:** Loss of balance or reaching out when trying to touch the elbow and knee, torso shifting sideways or otherwise moving.

Remember to score both sides.

PAIN CLEARANCE TEST 1. Kneel on the floor with your lower legs behind you.   **2.** Sit back on your heels.   **3.** Reach forward with your arms and try to put them and your head on the floor.

If you experience pain in your lower back, see your doctor.

FIXES

FIX 1: Bird Dog (page 182) done in a slow, controlled manner with normal breathing

FIX 2: Lower Body Rolling (page 185)

FIX 3: Upper Body Rolling (page 185)

PART 2
THE PROGRAMS

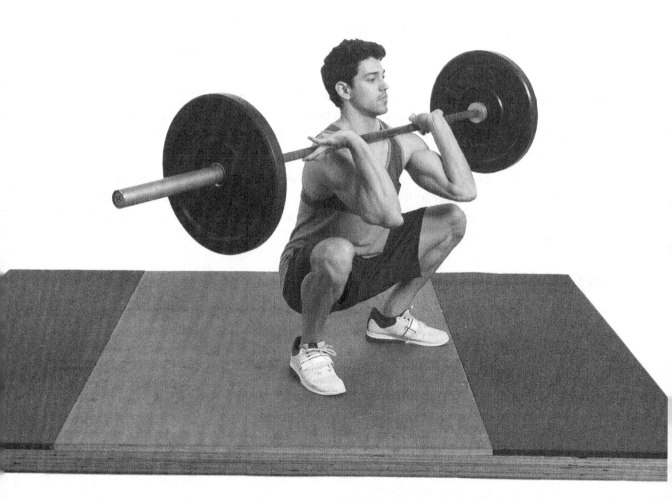

Learning the Olympic lifts may seem like a daunting task, but it's not. To help you start at whatever level you may be at, I've created a 12-week program divided into three 4-week phases. Each phase builds upon the prior phase. If you're a newbie, keep your training to the a minimum of 3 days per week. More advanced lifters who are in better shape can train 4–5 days per week, but make sure you're getting adequate rest. Rest/recovery days are just as important as the training, especially as you get older.

Please take your time going through the lifts. You may have been doing them for a while but it never hurts to practice the basics. Jumping the gun will not help you in the long run. Use PVC and an unweighted bar while you're learning the basics. After a few weeks, add a little weight to the bar. Remember, quality of movement is more important than quantity (reps or poundage).

Vary your training on the off days. If you find that the lifting workouts are demanding, ease up on your off-day training. On the other hand, if the lifting workouts are easy to moderate, then by all means take it up a notch on the other days.

Phase I focuses on practicing your technique. You'll work on the individual parts of the lifts for the first two weeks then start putting the pieces together the last two weeks.

Phase II continues the development and maintenance of good technique while slowly increasing the load, which is determined by the number of reps. You'll be using the bar and heavier weights that work in 3–5 sets of 3–5 reps. If you're doing sets of 5, the weight should be lower than if you're doing sets of 3. While 3x5 and 5x3 are the same total reps, you should lift more weight (intensity) when doing 5 sets of 3 than when doing 3 sets of 5.

In **Phase III** you'll use percentages based off of your estimated 1 rep max (1RM), or the maximum amount of weight you can lift with good form. Each lift has its own 1RM—your calculated 1RM will be different for the power clean, full clean, and jerk. Don't worry, I've included some guidelines on how to test your 1RM before starting this phase.

Congratulations! When you finish Phase III, you should be a good Olympic lifter—and gotten quite a bit stronger in the process. What's next? If you want to permanently integrate lifting into your fitness lifestyle, by all means continue working on the fixes and safely adding load. If you want to take your newfound skills to the next level and compete, you'll need to find a coach.

WARMING UP

Warming up is the process of getting your body moving, increasing blood flow through your body, increasing the temperature of your muscles a little so that they move more freely, and getting your heart rate up a little. It's preparation for the training you're about to do.

Incorporating the foam roller and other self-myofascial release techniques helps to increase the blood flow to your muscles and helps them to loosen up a little. Everyone should use a foam roller on the outsides of the thighs, mid- and upper back, and lats. However, most people shouldn't roll or stretch their hamstrings if they feel they're tight. "Tight" hamstrings are typically caused by tightness in other muscles that tip the pelvis forward into a condition called anterior pelvic tilt (APT). Tight hip flexors and psoas as well as weak hamstrings and glutes are the common culprits. If you sit all day, and most of us do, you probably have APT—even many athletes have APT. Proper training and warm-ups can help alleviate the problem.

Incorporating Self-Myofascial Release

I like using self-myofascial release (SMFR) for warm-up, while other coaches use it post-workout to help reduce soreness and undo the tension created by lifting weights. If you scored poorly on a particular area, you need to release that area. Do the following before and after if you have the time.

When rolling, you may come across some trigger points (knots in the muscles). Maintain your position, breathe, and relax, trying to get your brain to release the trigger point. The end result will be more freedom of movement.

1. Active Straight-Leg Raise

- Roll the glutes with a foam roller or a lacrosse ball.

- Roll the front of the thigh (quads).

2. Shoulders

- Roll a lacrosse or tennis ball on the pectoralis major and minor (chest); don't roll over breast tissue.

- Roll a lacrosse ball on the upper back, traps, shoulders, and between the shoulder blades (scapula) and spine. Never roll on the spine!

3. Rotary Stability

- Foam roll the lats.

- Roll a lacrosse ball on the outside of the shoulder blades.

- Roll a lacrosse ball on the glutes.

4. Trunk Stability

- Roll a lacrosse or tennis ball on the pectoralis major and minor (chest); don't roll over breast tissue.

- Roll a lacrosse ball on the upper back, traps, shoulders, and between the shoulder blades (scapula) and spine. Never roll on the spine!

5. Inline Lunge

- Roll a lacrosse ball under the butt and on the side of the hip.

- Roll a massage stick all the way around the lower leg. Don't roll the shin bone.

- Foam roll the front of the thigh (quads).

- Foam roll the inner thigh, especially near the knee.

6. Hurdle Step

- Roll a lacrosse ball under the butt and on the side of the hip.

- Roll a massage stick all the way around the lower leg. Don't roll the shin bone.

- Foam roll the front of the thigh (quads).

- Foam roll the inner thigh, especially near the knee.

7. Overhead Squat

- Foam roll the inner thigh.

- Foam roll the front of the thigh (quads).

- Roll a lacrosse ball under the foot.

- Roll a massage stick all the way around the lower leg. Don't roll the shin bone.

Incorporating Self-Assessments

As we discussed earlier, the self-assessments are based on the functional movement screen (FMS) system and are designed to see how you move through various patterns. These patterns are basic foundational movements. If you compensate or can't do them within the bounds of the FMS, you need to focus on the fixes so you don't make things worse or get injured. The FMS says don't load a dysfunctional pattern. Therefore, you need to work on clearing any failing scores or asymmetries you may have uncovered.

The order in which you clear the screen is not the same as the order you did the assessments. The fixes are done from the most basic or primitive patterns (Active Straight-Leg Raise, Shoulder Mobility) to the transitional patters (Rotary Stability, Trunk Stability Push-Up) to the "big three" (Overhead Squat, Hurdle Step, Inline Lunge), and that's how you should attack any issues.

Always start with the lowest screen you had trouble with. Based on the chart below, the Active Straight-Leg Raise (ASLR) is the easiest pattern to clear, while the Overhead Squat (OHS) is the most challenging. For example, if you failed the OHS and were asymmetrical on the ASLR and RS, you should do the fixes for the ASLR first. As that clears up, tackle the RS. Once everything else is clear, focus on the OHS. It should take you no more than 5 minutes to do the releases you need to do.

To refresh your memory, the self-assessments (page 28) are:

MOVEMENT SCREEN	ASSOCIATED MOVEMENTS	EXAMPLE EXERCISE
Active Straight-Leg Raise	hip-hinge patterns	Deadlift, Clean, Snatch
Shoulder Mobility	overhead movements	Push-Up, Bench Press, Get-Up
Rotary Stability	unilateral or rotational movement	power movements, Olympic lifts, running
Trunk Stability	anything that requires maintaining a neutral spine (plank, deadlift, squat, etc.)	Push-Up, Mountain Climber
Inline Lunge	running, jumping	Lunge, Split Squat, running
Hurdle Step	running, jumping	running, jumping
Overhead Squat	squat or lifting a weight overhead	Squat, overhead work

If you have pain during any of the screens or associated movements, go see a doctor to find out what's causing the problem. Olympic lifting requires total-body mobility, so if you lack mobility or stability in your core, hips, or shoulders, don't train the lifts until those issues are cleared up. That's why it's so important to do the self-assessments outlined in "Are You Ready to Olympic Lift?" (page 28) and the exercise fixes (page 169).

Fixes, Mobilization, & Activation

If you uncovered issues during your self-assessment, you need to do the fixes as part of your warm-ups. Start with the easiest pattern to clear (Active Straight-Leg Raise) and work to the most challenging (Overhead Squat). The screens build up as the table above shows. If you don't clear up the lower movements first, you'll never clear the higher ones.

As part of your warm-up sequence and after your foam-rolling session, work on the fixes (page 169) specific to your self-assessment. Choose two of the fixes for the lowest level you found issues with. For example, if you had problem with the Active Straight-Leg Raise and Rotary Stability, pick two of the fixes for each and do them after your foam-roller work. You can do these every day; the more often you do them, the sooner the issue should clear up. The straight-leg raise issue should clear within a few sessions; some people might clear it in just one. You may find that if you have problems with the Overhead Squat self-assessment, those issues will be gone once you clear up the lower-level patterns.

After the foam-roller work and the fixes, move on to the dynamic warm-up phase. The dynamic warm-ups are designed to get your blood flowing more; you might even break a light sweat. You'll be doing Turkish get-ups, box jumps, footwork drills, and other quick movements to get your body primed for the Olympic lifts.

PROGRAM NOTES

You'll be doing complexes and combos in some of the sessions. A **complex** is performing a specific number of reps of one exercise, then immediately using the same weight and no rest performing another movement for a specific number of reps. There can be two, three, or more exercises in a complex. Many people use complexes as conditioning, which is fine for low-skill-level movements, but for the Olympic lifts go a little heavier and keep the reps between 3 and 5. Here's an example of a complex:

In the example below, you perform 5 Snatch High Pulls then 5 Snatches from the Scarecrow with no rest between the reps. This is 1 set. You then rest 1 minute before you continue to the next set for a total of 5 sets.

Exercise	Set/Rep/Duration	Rest
Snatch High Pull, page 122 + Snatch from the Scarecrow, page 124	5x5	1m between sets

A **combo** is similar but you'll do 1 rep of a lift then 1 rep of another lift. You can combine 3–5 movements into a combo. You won't set the weight down until you've completed the specified number of reps through the combo. The clean and jerk by its nature is actually a three-movement combo exercise. You do 1 clean into a front squat, stand, then go into the jerk.

In the example below, you perform 1 Hang Power Snatch then 1 Overhead Squat 5 times with no rest between the reps. This is 1 set. You then rest 1 minute before you continue to the next set for a total of 3 sets.

Exercise	Set/Rep/Duration	Rest
Hang Power Snatch, page 130 → Overhead Squat, page 119	3x5	1m between sets

Complexes and combos must be sequenced properly so that they flow seamlessly from one movement to another. For example, going from the Snatch Grip High Pull from Hang to the Snatch Grip Deadlift to the Hang Snatch doesn't flow well. You'll want to change the order to what we have above.

The load for the complex will be lighter than for the combo because you'll be doing fewer reps of each lift in the combo.

In this book, we indicate a combo with "→" and a complex with "+" between lifts.

WORKOUT KEY	
TERM	**DESCRIPTION**
Exercise	what you'll be doing
Sets/Reps/Duration	how many (3 sets of 5 reps, for example) or how long you'll perform the exercise
Rest	how long you'll rest after performing the exercise for the specified number of reps or stated duration
Comments	specific instructions or information pertaining to the exercise or set/reps/duration
s	seconds; so 30s = 30 seconds
m	minutes; so 1m = 1 minute
3x20s	this means 3 reps of 20 seconds of work
20s:20s	this indicates the exercise is unilateral—you'll do 20 seconds of work on one side, switch and immediately do 20 seconds of work on the other side
r/l	In some cases we write "3 r/l" to indicate that you'll be doing 3 reps of an exercise on each side.
yd	yards
AMRAP	as many reps as possible
→	indicates a combo exercise
+	indicates a complex exercise

PHASE I: BEGINNER PROGRAM

If you've never done Olympic lifting before or have only been training them for a short time, start with this phase of the training cycle. It's designed to allow you to train your technique, and you don't need to use anything but a PVC or unweighted bar for the first couple of weeks (6 sessions). Practice the movements!

Even if you've been doing the Olympic lifts for more than a year, it's still a good idea to go back and work on the basics. The better your foundation, the better your higher-level movements will be. It's just like constructing a pyramid—build a wide, solid base and work your way up.

If you don't have kettlebells or heavy ropes, I urge you to get them. They're great tools and you can train with them on your off days if you feel like you need to train more than 3 days per week.

PHASE I: Week 1, Day 1			
WARM-UP			
Exercise	*Set/Rep/Duration*	*Rest*	*Comments*
Foam roller			see "Incorporating Self-Myofascial Release" guidelines, page 39
Fixes			see "Are You Ready to Olympic Lift?" on page 28 for the self-assessment fixes you should do
Kettlebell Turkish Get-Up, page 158	1x3 r/l	30–60s	alternate arms
Box Jump, page 149	3x10s	10s	
MAIN WORKOUT			
Exercise	*Set/Rep/Duration*	*Rest*	*Comments*
Clean-Grip Pull, page 121	5x5	30–60s between sets	use PVC or unweighted bar; this is the Snatch Pull with a clean grip
Clean-Grip High Pull, page 89	5x5	30–60s between sets	use PVC or unweighted bar
Scarecrow Clean, page 91	5x5	30–60s between sets	use PVC or unweighted bar
Barbell Front Squat, page 145	5x5	30–60s between sets	use PVC or unweighted bar
CONDITIONING			
do the following exercises as a circuit 4 times			
Exercise	*Set/Rep/Duration*	*Rest*	*Comments*
Burpee, page 161	20s	20s	
Split Squat/Lunge variation, page 150	20s:20s	20s	do most advanced variation (Split Squat, Forward Lunge, Reverse Lunge, or Jumping Lunge) you can with good form
Push-Up, page 153 / Spiderman Push-Up, page 153	20s	20s	do most advanced variation you can with good form
Side Plank, page 157	20s:20s	20s	

WARM-UP

Exercise	Set/Rep/Duration	Rest	Comments
Foam roller			see "Incorporating Self-Myofascial Release" guidelines, page 39
Fixes			see "Are You Ready to Olympic Lift?" on page 28 for the self-assessment fixes you should do
Bootstrapper, page 154	1x8	30s	
Skipping Forward, page 164	3x15s	15s between sets	
Fast Feet Drill, page 161	3x15s	15s between sets	move fast
Carioca, page 160	3x15s:15s	15s between sets	

MAIN WORKOUT

Exercise	Set/Rep/Duration	Rest	Comments
Snatch Pull, page page 121	5x5	30–60s between sets	use PVC or unweighted bar
Snatch High Pull, page 122	5x5	30–60s between sets	use PVC or unweighted bar
Snatch from the Scarecrow, page 124	5x5	30–60s between sets	use PVC or unweighted bar
Barbell Back Squat, page 145	5x5	30–60s between sets	use PVC or unweighted bar

CONDITIONING

do the following exercises as a circuit 4 times

Exercise	Set/Rep/Duration	Rest	Comments
Mountain Climber, page 162	20s	20s	
Inverted Row, page 155	20s	20s	
Bear Crawl, page 162	20s	20s	
Goblet Squat, page 146	20s	20s	

PHASE I: Week 1, Day 3

WARM-UP

Exercise	Set/Rep/Duration	Rest	Comments
Foam roller			see "Incorporating Self-Myofascial Release" guidelines, page 39
Fixes			see "Are You Ready to Olympic Lift?" on page 28 for the self-assessment fixes you should do
Quad Press, page 153 / Quad Hop, page 154	3x15s	15s	do whichever variation you can
Kettlebell Double Dead Clean, page 147	1x8	60s	light and easy, practice technique
1-Arm Kettlebell Dead Snatch, page 148	1x8 r/l		light and easy, practice technique

MAIN WORKOUT

Exercise	Set/Rep/Duration	Rest	Comments
Press from Behind the Neck, page 108	5x5	30–60s between sets	use PVC or unweighted bar
Push Press from Behind the Neck, page 110	5x5	30–60s between sets	use PVC or unweighted bar
Power Jerk from Behind the Neck, page 113	5x5	30–60s between sets	use PVC or unweighted bar; no foot movement
Overhead Squat, page 119	5x5	30–60s between sets	use PVC or unweighted bar

CONDITIONING
do the following exercises as a circuit 4 times

Exercise	Set/Rep/Duration	Rest	Comments
Double Wave, page 165	20s	20s	
Alternating Waves, page 166	20s	20s	
In/Out Waves, page 166	20s	20s	

PHASE I: Week 2, Day 1

WARM-UP

Exercise	Set/Rep/Duration	Rest	Comments
Foam roller			see "Incorporating Self-Myofascial Release" guidelines, page 39
Fixes			see "Are You Ready to Olympic Lift?" on page 28 for the self-assessment fixes you should do
Kettlebell Turkish Get-Up, page 158	1x4 r/l		alternate arms each rep
Box Jump, page 149	3x15s	15s	

MAIN WORKOUT

Exercise	Set/Rep/Duration	Rest	Comments
Clean-Grip Pull, page 121	3x8	1m between sets	this is the Snatch Pull with a clean grip
Clean-Grip High Pull, page 89	3x8	1m between sets	
Scarecrow Clean, page 91	3x8	1m between sets	
Barbell Front Squat, page 145	3x8	1m between sets	

CONDITIONING
do the following exercises as a circuit 4 times

Exercise	Set/Rep/Duration	Rest	Comments
Burpee, page 161	20s	10s	
Split Squat/Lunge variation, page 150	20s:20s	10s	do most advanced variation (Split Squat, Forward Lunge, Reverse Lunge, or Jumping Lunge) you can with good form
Push-Up, page 153 / Spiderman Push-Up, page 153	20s	10s	do most advanced variation you can with good form
Side Plank, page 157	20s:20s	10s	

PHASE I: Week 2, Day 2

WARM-UP

Exercise	Set/Rep/Duration	Rest	Comments
Foam roller			see "Incorporating Self-Myofascial Release" guidelines, page 39
Fixes			see "Are You Ready to Olympic Lift?" on page 28 for the self-assessment fixes you should do
Bootstrapper, page 154	1x10		
Skipping Forward, page 164	3x20s	10s	
Fast Feet Drill, page 161	3x20s	10s	
Carioca, page 160	3x20s:20s	10s	

MAIN WORKOUT

Exercise	Set/Rep/Duration	Rest	Comments
Snatch Pull, page 121	3x8	1m between sets	
Snatch High Pull, page 122	3x8	1m between sets	
Snatch from the Scarecrow, page 124	3x8	1m between sets	
Barbell Back Squat, page 145	3x8	1m between sets	

CONDITIONING

do the following exercises as a circuit 4 times

Exercise	Set/Rep/Duration	Rest	Comments
Mountain Climber, page 162	20s	10s	
Inverted Row, page 155	20s	10s	
Bear Crawl, page 162	20s	10s	
Goblet Squat, page 146	20s	10s	

WARM-UP

Exercise	Set/Rep/Duration	Rest	Comments
Foam roller			see "Incorporating Self-Myofascial Release" guidelines, page 39
Fixes			see "Are You Ready to Olympic Lift?" on page 28 for the self-assessment fixes you should do
Quad Press, page 153 / Quad Hop, page 154	1x20s	20s	
Kettlebell Double Dead Clean, page 147	1x10		use light weight
1-Arm Kettlebell Dead Snatch, page 148	1x10 r/l		use light weight

MAIN WORKOUT

Exercise	Set/Rep/Duration	Rest	Comments
Press from Behind the Neck, page 108	3x8		
Push Press from Behind the Neck, page 110	3x8	1m between sets	
Power Jerk from Behind the Neck, page 113	3x8	1m between sets	no foot movement
Overhead Squat, page 119	3x8	1m between sets	

CONDITIONING

do the following exercises as a circuit 4 times

Exercise	Set/Rep/Duration	Rest	Comments
Double Wave, page 165	20s	10s	
Alternating Waves, page 166	20s	10s	
In/Out Waves, page 166	20s	10s	

PHASE I: Week 3, Day 1

WARM-UP

Exercise	Set/Rep/Duration	Rest	Comments
Foam roller			see "Incorporating Self-Myofascial Release" guidelines, page 39
Fixes			see "Are You Ready to Olympic Lift?" on page 28 for the self-assessment fixes you should do
Kettlebell Turkish Get-Up, page 158	1x5 r/l		alternate arms each rep
Box Jump, page 149	3x20s	10s	

MAIN WORKOUT

Exercise	Set/Rep/Duration	Rest	Comments
Muscle High Pull, page 87 + Scarecrow Clean, page 91	5x5	1m between sets	complex
Clean-Grip Conventional Deadlift, page 142	5x5	1m between sets	
Barbell Front Squat, page 145	5x5	1m between sets	

CONDITIONING
do the following exercises as a circuit 4 times

Exercise	Set/Rep/Duration	Rest	Comments
Burpee, page 161	30s	30s	
Split Squat/Lunge variation, page 150	30s:30s	30s	do most advanced variation (Split Squat, Forward Lunge, Reverse Lunge, or Jumping Lunge) you can with good form
Push-Up, page 153 / Spiderman Push-Up, page 153	30s	30s	do most advanced variation you can with good form
Side Plank, page 157	30s:30s	30s	

PHASE I: Week 3, Day 2

WARM-UP

Exercise	Set/Rep/Duration	Rest	Comments
Foam roller			see "Incorporating Self-Myofascial Release" guidelines, page 39
Fixes			see "Are You Ready to Olympic Lift?" on page 28 for the self-assessment fixes you should do
Bootstrapper, page 154	1x10		
Skipping Forward, page 164	3x30s	15s	
Fast Feet Drill, page 161	3x30s	15s	
Carioca, page 160	3x30s:30s	15s	

MAIN WORKOUT

Exercise	Set/Rep/Duration	Rest	Comments
Snatch High Pull, page 122 + Snatch from the Scarecrow, page 124	5x5	1m between sets	complex
Snatch-Grip Conventional Deadlift, page 142	5x5	1m between sets	
Snatch-Grip Barbell Overhead Squat, page 119	5x5	1m between sets	

CONDITIONING
do the following exercises as a circuit 4 times

Exercise	Set/Rep/Duration	Rest	Comments
Mountain Climber, page 162	30s	30s	
Inverted Row, page 155	30s	30s	
Bear Crawl, page 162	30s	30s	
Goblet Squat, page 146	30s	30s	

PHASE I: Week 3, Day 3

WARM-UP

Exercise	Set/Rep/Duration	Rest	Comments
Foam roller			see "Incorporating Self-Myofascial Release" guidelines, page 39
Fixes			see "Are You Ready to Olympic Lift?" on page 28 for the self-assessment fixes you should do
Quad Press, page 153 / Quad Hop, page 154	1x30s	15s	
Kettlebell Double Dead Clean, page 147	1x6		use moderate weight
1-Arm Kettlebell Dead Snatch, page 148	1x6 r/l		use moderate weight

MAIN WORKOUT

Exercise	Set/Rep/Duration	Rest	Comments
Push Press, page 111	5x5	1m between sets	
Split Jerk, page 115	5x5	1m between sets	
Barbell Back Squat, page 145	5x5	1m between sets	

CONDITIONING
do the following exercises as a circuit 4 times

Exercise	Set/Rep/Duration	Rest	Comments
Double Wave, page 165	30s	30s	
Alternating Waves, page 166	30s	30s	
In/Out Waves, page 166	30s	30s	

WARM-UP

Exercise	Set/Rep/Duration	Rest	Comments
Foam roller			see "Incorporating Self-Myofascial Release" guidelines, page 39
Fixes			see "Are You Ready to Olympic Lift?" on page 28 for the self-assessment fixes you should do
Kettlebell Turkish Get-Up, page 158	1x3 r/l		do NOT switch arms per rep
Box Jump, page 149	2x30s	15s	

MAIN WORKOUT

Exercise	Set/Rep/Duration	Rest	Comments
High Pull, page 89 + Hang Power Clean, page 94	5x5	1m between sets	complex
Hang Power Clean, page 94 + Barbell Front Squat, page 145	5x5	1m between sets	complex
Halting Deadlift, page 128	5x5		

CONDITIONING

do the clean and squats as a circuit 3 times, rest 1 minute, then do the farmer's walk

Exercise	Set/Rep/Duration	Rest	Comments
Kettlebell Double Dead Clean, page 147	8	none between cleans and the squats	
Double Kettlebell Front Squat, page 147	8	1m before Farmer's Walk	
Double Farmer's Walk, page 167	3 x 20yd	30s between sets	

WARM-UP

Exercise	Set/Rep/Duration	Rest	Comments
Foam roller			see "Incorporating Self-Myofascial Release" guidelines, page 39
Fixes			see "Are You Ready to Olympic Lift?" on page 28 for the self-assessment fixes you should do
Bootstrapper, page 154	1x10		
Skipping Forward, page 164	3x30s	15s	
Fast Feet Drill, page 161	3x30s	15s	
Carioca, page 160	3x30s:30s	15s	

MAIN WORKOUT

Exercise	Set/Rep/Duration	Rest	Comments
Snatch High Pull, page 122 + Hang Power Snatch, page 130	5x5	1m between sets	complex
Hang Power Snatch, page 130 + Barbell Overhead Squat, page 119	5x5	1m between sets	complex
Snatch First Pull, page 126	5x5	1m between sets	

CONDITIONING

do the first 2 exercises as a circuit 3 times then do the plank circuit 1 time

Exercise	Set/Rep/Duration	Rest	Comments
1-Arm Kettlebell Dead Snatch, page 148	10 r/l	none between arms; 30s before pull-ups	use moderate weight
Pull-Up, page 154	AMRAP	rest 1m	strict, no kipping
Plank Circuit			
Forearm Plank, page 156	1m	no rest	
Raise right arm only	15s	no rest	
Raise left arm only	15s	no rest	
Raise right leg only	15s	no rest	
Raise left leg only	15s	no rest	
Raise right arm and left leg only	15s	no rest	
Raise left arm and right leg only	15s	no rest	
Side Plank right side, page 157	15s	no rest	
Side Plank left side, page 157	15s	no rest	
Forearm Plank, page 156	1m	no rest	

PHASE I: Week 4, Day 3

WARM-UP

Exercise	Set/Rep/Duration	Rest	Comments
Foam roller			see "Incorporating Self-Myofascial Release" guidelines, page 39
Fixes			see "Are You Ready to Olympic Lift?" on page 28 for the self-assessment fixes you should do
Quad Press, page 153 / Quad Hop, page 154	1x30s	15s	
Kettlebell Double Dead Clean, page 147	1x6		use moderate weight
1-Arm Kettlebell Dead Snatch, page 148	1x6 r/l		use moderate weight

MAIN WORKOUT

Exercise	Set/Rep/Duration	Rest	Comments
Split Jerk, page 115	3x5		
Hang Power Clean, page 94 + Split Jerk, page 115	3x5		complex
Clean First Pull, page 98	3x5		

CONDITIONING
do the following exercises as a circuit 4 times

Exercise	Set/Rep/Duration	Rest	Comments
Super Plank, page 156	20s	20s	
1-Arm Farmer's Walk, page 167 + 1-Arm Rack Walk, page 167	20yd then switch arms		complex
Split Squat/Lunge variation, page 150	20s:20s	20s	do most advanced variation (Split Squat, Forward Lunge, Reverse Lunge, or Jumping Lunge) you can with good form

PHASE II: INTERMEDIATE PROGRAM

Congratulations! By now you should have a pretty good grasp of the Olympic lifts and are ready to work on refining your technique and adding more weight to the bar. Don't go too heavy too soon, though. Doing so will keep you from perfecting your form. Just because you can do a heavy jerk or snatch doesn't mean you should, especially if you have to use bad form to get it up! Remember, safety first.

Going into Phase II, you'll be dropping the reps to 5 or 6 max and working on combinations and complexes. These are just ways of combining movements to reinforce technique or to work on weak sections of a lift. Complexes and combos are more intense so you'll want to err on the side of caution and use moderate loads. You'll also be ramping up on the conditioning portion of your workouts, too, as you want to increase your cardio and develop or maintain your athleticism through a variety of movements and equipment.

PHASE II: Week 1, Day 1			
WARM-UP			
Exercise	*Set/Rep/Duration*	*Rest*	*Comments*
Foam roller			see "Incorporating Self-Myofascial Release" guidelines, page 39
Fixes			see "Are You Ready to Olympic Lift?" on page 28 for the self-assessment fixes you should do
Arm Bar, page 173	1x30s:30s		use light bell or no weight
Half Get-Up, page 158	1x5 r/l		perform Turkish Get-Up until seated position, then return to the floor; use light bell or no weight
Fast Feet Drill, page 161	3x20s	10s	if this is getting easy, raise the step up a little
MAIN WORKOUT			
Exercise	*Set/Rep/Duration*	*Rest*	*Comments*
Hang Power Clean, page 94 → Barbell Front Squat, page 145	3x5	1m between sets	combo
Clean-Grip Halting Deadlift, page 128	3x5	1m between sets	
High Pull from the Floor	3x5	1m between sets	this is a combination of the First Pull (page 98) and High Pull (page 89)
CONDITIONING			
do the following exercises as a circuit 4 times			
Exercise	*Set/Rep/Duration*	*Rest*	*Comments*
Double Kettlebell Front Squat, page 147	10	no rest	
1-Arm Farmer's Walk, page 167	20yd r/l	no rest	
Push-Up, page 153 / Spiderman Push-Up, page 153	AMRAP	rest 1m	do most advanced variation you can with good form

PHASE II: Week 1, Day 2

WARM-UP

Exercise	Set/Rep/Duration	Rest	Comments
Foam roller			see "Incorporating Self-Myofascial Release" guidelines, page 39
Fixes			see "Are You Ready to Olympic Lift?" on page 28 for the self-assessment fixes you should do
Skipping Forward, page 164	3x15s	10s	
Side Shuffle, page 164	3x15s:15s	10s	
Carioca, page 160	3x15s:15s	10s	

MAIN WORKOUT

Exercise	Set/Rep/Duration	Rest	Comments
Hang Power Snatch, page 130 → Overhead Squat, page 119	3x5	1m between sets	combo
Snatch-Grip Halting Deadlift, page 128	3x5	1m between sets	
Snatch-Grip High Pull from Floor	3x5	1m between sets	this is a combination of the Snatch First Pull (page 126) and Snatch High Pull (page 122)

CONDITIONING
do the following exercises as a circuit 3 times

Exercise	Set/Rep/Duration	Rest	Comments
Kettlebell Double Dead Clean, page 147	30s	15s	
Double Wave, page 165	30s	15s	
1-Arm Kettlebell Dead Snatch, page 148	30s:30s	15s	
Alternating Waves, page 166	30s	30s	

PHASE II: Week 1, Day 3

WARM-UP

Exercise	Set/Rep/Duration	Rest	Comments
Foam roller			see "Incorporating Self-Myofascial Release" guidelines, page 39
Fixes			see "Are You Ready to Olympic Lift?" on page 28 for the self-assessment fixes you should do
Kettlebell Turkish Get-Up, page 158	1x3 r/l		
Quad Press, page 153	3x15s	15s	

MAIN WORKOUT

Exercise	Set/Rep/Duration	Rest	Comments
Hang Power Clean, page 94 → Press, page 109	3x5	1m between sets	combo
Hang Power Clean, page 94 → Push Press, page 111	3x5	1m between sets	combo
Hang Power Clean, page 94 → Split Jerk, page 115	3x5	1m between sets	combo
Barbell Back Squat, page 145	3x5	1m between sets	

CONDITIONING

do the following exercises as a circuit 4 times

Exercise	Set/Rep/Duration	Rest	Comments
Bottom's-Up Walk, page 168	20yd r/l	minimal rest	use light to moderate weight
Inverted Row, page 155	10	minimal rest	explosive on the pull, slow on the lowering
Barbell Hip Thruster, page 179	12		don't go too heavy: women start with 95lbs, guys 135lbs. If it's really easy, go up 10lbs on each set until it's challenging

PHASE II: Week 2, Day 1

WARM-UP

Exercise	Set/Rep/Duration	Rest	Comments
Foam roller			see "Incorporating Self-Myofascial Release" guidelines, page 39
Fixes			see "Are You Ready to Olympic Lift?" on page 28 for the self-assessment fixes you should do
Arm Bar, page 173	1x5 r/l		
Half Get-Up, page 158	1x5 r/l		perform Turkish Get-Up until seated position, then return to the floor
Fast Feet Drill, page 161	3x20s	10s	

MAIN WORKOUT

Exercise	Set/Rep/Duration	Rest	Comments
Clean First Pull, page 98 → Hang Power Clean, page 94	3x5		combo
Barbell Front Squat, page 145 → Barbell Push Press, page 111	5x5		combo; use light weight
Clean-Grip Romanian Deadlift, page 143	3x5	1m between sets	

CONDITIONING
do the following exercises as a circuit 4 times

Exercise	Set/Rep/Duration	Rest	Comments
Double Kettlebell Front Squat, page 147	8	minimal rest	
1-Arm Farmer's Walk, page 167	30yd r/l	minimal rest	
Push-Up, page 153 / Spiderman Push-Up, page 153	AMRAP	minimal rest	do most advanced variation you can with good form

PHASE II: Week 2, Day 2

WARM-UP

Exercise	Set/Rep/Duration	Rest	Comments
Foam roller			see "Incorporating Self-Myofascial Release" guidelines, page 39
Fixes			see "Are You Ready to Olympic Lift?" on page 28 for the self-assessment fixes you should do
Skipping Forward, page 164	3x15s	10s	
Side Shuffle, page 164	3x15s	10s	
Carioca, page 160	3x15s	10s	

MAIN WORKOUT

Exercise	Set/Rep/Duration	Rest	Comments
Snatch First Pull, page 126 → Hang Power Snatch, page 130	3x5	1m between sets	combo (pause between the 2 exercises)
Barbell Back Squat, page 145 → Sots Press, page 146	5x5	1m between sets	combo; light weight
Snatch-Grip Romanian Deadlift, page 143	3x5	1m between sets	

CONDITIONING
do the following exercises as a circuit 3 times

Exercise	Set/Rep/Duration	Rest	Comments
Kettlebell Double Dead Clean, page 147	40s	20s	use moderate weight
Double Wave, page 165	40s	20s	fast!
1-Arm Kettlebell Dead Snatch, page 148	40s:40s	20s	use moderate weight
Alternating Waves, page 166	40s	20s	fast!

PHASE II: Week 2, Day 3

WARM-UP

Exercise	Set/Rep/Duration	Rest	Comments
Foam roller			see "Incorporating Self-Myofascial Release" guidelines, page 39
Fixes			see "Are You Ready to Olympic Lift?" on page 28 for the self-assessment fixes you should do
Kettlebell Turkish Get-Up, page 158	1x3 r/l		
Quad Press, page 153	3x15s	15s	

MAIN WORKOUT

Exercise	Set/Rep/Duration	Rest	Comments
Hang Power Clean, page 94 → Split Jerk, page 115	3x5	1m between sets	combo
Press from Behind the Neck, page 108	5x5	1m between sets	
Overhead Squat, page 119	3x5	1m between sets	

CONDITIONING
do the following exercises as a circuit 3 times

Exercise	Set/Rep/Duration	Rest	Comments
Bottom's-Up Walk, page 168	30yd r/l	minimal rest	use light to moderate weight
Inverted Row, page 155	12	minimal rest	explosive pull, slow release
Barbell Hip Thruster, page 179	15	minimal rest	use the same weight you finished with the last time you did these

PHASE II: Week 3, Day 1

WARM-UP

Exercise	Set/Rep/Duration	Rest	Comments
Foam roller			see "Incorporating Self-Myofascial Release" guidelines, page 39
Fixes			see "Are You Ready to Olympic Lift?" on page 28 for the self-assessment fixes you should do
Kettlebell Turkish Get-Up, page 158	1x5 r/l		
Box Jump, page 149	3x15s	15s	

MAIN WORKOUT

Exercise	Set/Rep/Duration	Rest	Comments
Power Clean from Floor, page 103	3x5	1–2m between sets	
Barbell Front Squat, page 145	3x5	1–2m between sets	
Behind-the-Neck Split Jerk, page 115	3x5	1–2m between sets	

CONDITIONING
do the following exercises as a circuit 3 times

Exercise	Set/Rep/Duration	Rest	Comments
Double Kettlebell Front Squat, page 147	6	minimal rest	
1-Arm Farmer's Walk, page 167	40yd r/l	minimal rest	
Push-Up, page 153 / Spiderman Push-Up, page 153	AMRAP	minimal rest	do most advanced variation you can with good form

PHASE II: Week 3, Day 2

WARM-UP

Exercise	Set/Rep/Duration	Rest	Comments
Foam roller			see "Incorporating Self-Myofascial Release" guidelines, page 39
Fixes			see "Are You Ready to Olympic Lift?" on page 28 for the self-assessment fixes you should do
Quad Press, page 153	3x20s	20s	
Kettlebell Double Dead Clean, page 147	2x8	30s between sets	use moderate weight

MAIN WORKOUT

Exercise	Set/Rep/Duration	Rest	Comments
Power Snatch from the Floor, page 133	3x5	1–2m between sets	
Overhead Squat, page 119	3x5	1–2m between sets	
Snatch-Grip Conventional Deadlift, page 142	3x5	1–2m between sets	

CONDITIONING
do the following exercises as a circuit 4 times

Exercise	Set/Rep/Duration	Rest	Comments
Kettlebell Double Dead Clean, page 147	20s	10s	use heavy weight
Double Wave, page 165	20s	10s	fast!
1-Arm Kettlebell Dead Snatch, page 148	20s:20s	10s	use heavy weight
Alternating Waves, page 166	20s	10s	fast!

PHASE II: Week 3, Day 3

WARM-UP

Exercise	Set/Rep/Duration	Rest	Comments
Foam roller			see "Incorporating Self-Myofascial Release" guidelines, page 39
Fixes			see "Are You Ready to Olympic Lift?" on page 28 for the self-assessment fixes you should do
1-Arm Kettlebell Dead Snatch, page 148	2x8 r/l		
Bear Crawl, page 162 / Spiderman Crawl, page 163	2x15s	15s	do most advanced variation you can with good form

MAIN WORKOUT

Exercise	Set/Rep/Duration	Rest	Comments
Hang Clean, page 96 → Split Jerk, page 115 OR Hang Power Clean, page 94 → Split Jerk, page 115	3x5	1–2m between sets	combo; if you can't get rock bottom, do a Hang Power Clean
Clean-Grip Conventional Deadlift, page 142	3x5	1–2m between sets	
Snatch High Pull, page 122	3x5	1–2m between sets	

CONDITIONING
do the following exercises as a circuit 4 times

Exercise	Set/Rep/Duration	Rest	Comments
Bottom's-Up Walk, page 168	40yd r/l	minimal rest between exercises	
Inverted Row, page 155	8	minimal rest between exercises	
Barbell Hip Thruster, page 179	15	minimal rest between exercises	

PHASE II: Week 4, Day 1

WARM-UP

Exercise	Set/Rep/Duration	Rest	Comments
Foam roller			see "Incorporating Self-Myofascial Release" guidelines, page 39
Fixes			see "Are You Ready to Olympic Lift?" on page 28 for the self-assessment fixes you should do
Arm Bar, page 173	1x5 r/l		
Half Get-Up, page 158	1x5 r/l		perform Turkish Get-Up until seated position, then return to the floor
Fast Feet Drill, page 161	3x20s	10s	

MAIN WORKOUT

Exercise	Set/Rep/Duration	Rest	Comments
Clean, page 104	5x3	2m between sets	use heavy weight

CONDITIONING
do the following exercises as a circuit 3 times

Exercise	Set/Rep/Duration	Rest	Comments
Bear Crawl, page 162 / Spiderman Crawl, page 163	30yd		do most advanced variation you can with good form
Split Squat/Lunge variation, page 150	30s:30s	30s	do most advanced variation (Split Squat, Forward Lunge, Reverse Lunge, or Jumping Lunge) you can with good form
Kettlebell Double Dead Clean, page 147	30s	30s	

PHASE II: Week 4, Day 2

WARM-UP

Exercise	Set/Rep/Duration	Rest	Comments
Foam roller			see "Incorporating Self-Myofascial Release" guidelines, page 39
Fixes			see "Are You Ready to Olympic Lift?" on page 28 for the self-assessment fixes you should do
Skipping Forward, page 164	3x15s	10s	
Side Shuffle, page 164	3x15s:15s	10s	
Carioca, page 160	3x15s:15s	10s	

MAIN WORKOUT

Exercise	Set/Rep/Duration	Rest	Comments
Snatch, page 138	5x3	2m between sets	use heavy weight

CONDITIONING

do the following exercises as a circuit 4 times

Exercise	Set/Rep/Duration	Rest	Comments
Double Farmer's Walk, page 167	40yd		
Double Kettlebell Dead Snatch, page 148	10		
Super Plank, page 156	AMRAP		

PHASE II: Week 4, Day 3

WARM-UP

Exercise	Set/Rep/Duration	Rest	Comments
Foam roller			see "Incorporating Self-Myofascial Release" guidelines, page 39
Fixes			see "Are You Ready to Olympic Lift?" on page 28 for the self-assessment fixes you should do
Kettlebell Turkish Get-Up, page 158	1x3 r/l		
Quad Press, page 153	3x15s	15s	

MAIN WORKOUT

Exercise	Set/Rep/Duration	Rest	Comments
Clean & Jerk	5x3	2m between sets	this is a combination of the Full Clean from the Floor (page 104) followed by the Split Jerk (page 115); use heavy weight

CONDITIONING
do the following exercises as a circuit 4 times

Exercise	Set/Rep/Duration	Rest	Comments
Double Wave, page 165	40s	20s	
Alternating Waves, page 166	40s	20s	
In/Out Waves, page 166	40s	20s	

PHASE III: ADVANCED PROGRAM

Now that you've successfully finished Phase II, it's time to start working with heavier weights. Phase III requires you to determine your 1 rep max (1RM) because the workouts in this phase are based on a percentages of your 1RM.

Determining Your 1 Rep Max

Once you've gotten your form in good shape with Phase II of the 12-week program, you'll need to determine your 1 rep max (RM), which is how much weight you can lift one time with good form. Your programming in Phase III will be based on percentages of your 1RM. Doing 5 reps at 50% 1RM will have a much different impact on your body than 5 reps at 80–90% of 1RM.

You'll need to determine your 1RM in the hang power clean (HPC), power clean (PC) from the floor, full clean, split jerk, and clean and jerk, as well as the full snatch, hang power snatch (HPS), power snatch (PS) from the floor, and the overhead squat (OHS). *Do not do all of these in one day!*

1. Warm up thoroughly to get your blood flowing with your foam roller, your fixes, and some easy box jumps.

2. Start with Hang Power Cleans. Load up with the poundage you've been working with and do 5 reps.

3. Rest 2 minutes.

4. Add 10 pounds to the bar and perform 5 reps.

5. If you did all 5 with good form, rest 5 minutes, and add 5–10 pounds, and repeat until you can no longer get 5 good reps.

Once you've failed to get a good set of 5, add 5 pounds to that weight and use that as your 1RM.

Over the course of 5 days, use this same procedure for all the other lifts.

Use the chart below to track your poundage:

	LIFT	ATTEMPT 1	ATTEMPT 2	ATTEMPT 3	ATTEMPT 4	1RM*
DAY 1	Hang Power Clean, page 94					
DAY 1	Split Jerk, page 115 (with squat rack or jerk blocks)					
DAY 2	Clean, page 104					
DAY 2	Power Clean from the Floor, page 103					
DAY 3	Clean & Jerk, page 104 + page 115					
DAY 3	Overhead Squat, page 119					
DAY 4	Hang Power Snatch, page 130					
DAY 4	Power Snatch from the Floor, page 133					
DAY 5	Snatch, page 138					

* add 5 pounds to attempt you didn't get 5 good reps

Periodically (typically every 4–6 weeks) you'll need to re-check your 1RMs. Re-testing will show whether you're getting stronger. If you're not making gains, you may have overestimated your current 1RM or are undertraining or overtraining. On the other hand, your technique may be off a bit, but without a coach you won't know for sure. If you feel that your technique is off, go back through the first two phases using heavier weights and hone your technique. That goes for everyone, not just beginners.

PHASE III: Week 1, Day 1

WARM-UP

Exercise	Set/Rep/Duration	Rest	Comments
Foam roller			See "Incorporating Self-Myofascial Release" guidelines, page 39
Fixes			see "Are You Ready to Olympic Lift?" on page 28 for the self-assessment fixes you should do
Fast Feet Drill, page 161	3x10s	5s	
Side Shuffle, page 164	3x10s:10s	10s	
Bootstrapper, page 154	1x45s		

MAIN WORKOUT

Exercise	Set/Rep/Duration	Rest	Comments
Hang Power Clean, page 94	1x5 @50% 1RM	1–2m	warm-up set
	1x3 @60% 1RM	1–2m	warm-up set
	3x3 @80% 1RM	2m between sets	The Real Work
Barbell Front Squat, page 145	3x3	2m between sets	go heavy
Press, page 109	3x3	2m between sets	go heavy

CONDITIONING
do the following exercises as a circuit 3 times

Exercise	Set/Rep/Duration	Rest	Comments
Double Kettlebell Front Squat, page 147	30s	30s	
Burpee, page 161	30s	30s	
Side Plank, page 157	30s:30s	60s	

PHASE III: Week 1, Day 2

WARM-UP

Exercise	Set/Rep/Duration	Rest	Comments
Foam roller			see "Incorporating Self-Myofascial Release" guidelines, page 39
Fixes			see "Are You Ready to Olympic Lift?" on page 28 for the self-assessment fixes you should do
Kettlebell Turkish Get-Up, page 158	1x5 r/l		
Box Jump, page 149	1x12		
Carioca, page 160	3x15s:15s		

MAIN WORKOUT

Exercise	Set/Rep/Duration	Rest	Comments
Hang Power Snatch, page 130	1x5 @50% 1RM	1–2m	warm-up set
	1x3 @60% 1RM	1–2m	warm-up set
	3x3 @80% 1RM	2m between sets	The Real Work
Overhead Squat, page 119	3x3	2m between sets	go heavy
Push Press, page 111	3x3	2m between sets	go heavy

CONDITIONING
do the following exercises as a circuit 4 times

Exercise	Set/Rep/Duration	Rest	Comments
Double Kettlebell Dead Snatch, page 148	30s	30s	
Mountain Climber, page 162	30s	30s	
Alternating Waves, page 166	30s	60s	

PHASE III: Week 1, Day 3

WARM-UP

Exercise	Set/Rep/Duration	Rest	Comments
Foam roller			see "Incorporating Self-Myofascial Release" guidelines, page 39
Fixes			see "Are You Ready to Olympic Lift?" on page 28 for the self-assessment fixes you should do
Bear Crawl, page 162 / Spiderman Crawl, page 163	2x30s	30s	do most advanced variation you can with good form
Half Get-Up, page 158	1x5 r/l		perform Turkish Get-Up until seated position, then return to the floor
Split Squat/Lunge variation, page 150	2x30s:30s	30s	do most advanced variation (Split Squat, Forward Lunge, Reverse Lunge, or Jumping Lunge) you can with good form

MAIN WORKOUT

Exercise	Set/Rep/Duration	Rest	Comments
Hang Power Clean, page 94 → Split Jerk, page 115	1x5 @50% 1RM	1–2m	combo; warm-up set
	1x3 @60% 1RM	1–2m	warm-up set
	3x3 @75% 1RM	2m between sets	The Real Work
Snatch-Grip Conventional Deadlift, page 142	3x3	2m between sets	go heavy

CONDITIONING
do the following exercises as a circuit 4 times

Exercise	Set/Rep/Duration	Rest	Comments
Super Plank, page 156	30s	30s	
Goblet Squat, page 146	30s	30s	
Inverted Row, page 155	30s	30s	

WARM-UP

Exercise	Set/Rep/Duration	Rest	Comments
Foam roller			See "Incorporating Self-Myofascial Release" guidelines, page 39
Fixes			see "Are You Ready to Olympic Lift?" on page 28 for the self-assessment fixes you should do
Fast Feet Drill, page 161	3x10s	5s	
Side Shuffle, page 164	3x10s:10s	10s	
Bootstrapper, page 154	1x45s		

MAIN WORKOUT

Exercise	Set/Rep/Duration	Rest	Comments
Clean, page 104	1x5 @50% 1RM	1–2m	warm-up set
	1x3 @60% 1RM	1–2m	warm-up set
	3x3 @80% 1RM	2m between sets	
Barbell Front Squat, page 145	3x5	2m between sets	go heavy
Press, page 109	3x5	2m between sets	go heavy

CONDITIONING

do the following exercises as a circuit 3 times

Exercise	Set/Rep/Duration	Rest	Comments
Double Kettlebell Front Squat, page 147	30s	15s	
Burpee, page 161	30s	15s	
Side Plank, page 157	30s:30s	60s	

PHASE III: Week 2, Day 2

WARM-UP

Exercise	Set/Rep/Duration	Rest	Comments
Foam roller			see "Incorporating Self-Myofascial Release" guidelines, page 39
Fixes			see "Are You Ready to Olympic Lift?" on page 28 for the self-assessment fixes you should do
Kettlebell Turkish Get-Up, page 158	1x5 r/l		
Box Jump, page 149	1x12		
Carioca, page 160	3x15s:15s	15s	

MAIN WORKOUT

Exercise	Set/Rep/Duration	Rest	Comments
Snatch, page 138	1x5 @50% 1RM	1–2m	warm-up set
	1x3 @60% 1RM	1–2m	warm-up set
	3x3 @80% 1RM	2m between sets	
Overhead Squat, page 119	3x5	2m between sets	go heavy
Push Press, page 111	3x5	2m between sets	go heavy

CONDITIONING
do the following exercises as a circuit 4 times

Exercise	Set/Rep/Duration	Rest	Comments
Double Kettlebell Dead Snatch, page 148	30s	15s	
Mountain Climber, page 162	30s	15s	
Alternating Waves, page 166	30s	60s	

WARM-UP

Exercise	Set/Rep/Duration	Rest	Comments
Foam roller			see "Incorporating Self-Myofascial Release" guidelines, page 39
Fixes			see "Are You Ready to Olympic Lift?" on page 28 for the self-assessment fixes you should do
Bear Crawl, page 162 / Spiderman Crawl, page 163	2x30s	30s	do most advanced variation you can with good form
Half Get-Up, page 158	1x5 r/l		perform Turkish Get-Up until seated position, then return to the floor
Split Squat/Lunge variation, page 150	2x30s:30s	30s	do most advanced variation (Split Squat, Forward Lunge, Reverse Lunge, or Jumping Lunge) you can with good form

MAIN WORKOUT

Exercise	Set/Rep/Duration	Rest	Comments
Clean & Jerk	1x5 @50% 1RM	1–2m	this is a combination of the Full Clean from the Floor (page 104) followed by the Split Jerk (page 115); warm-up set
	1x3 @60% 1RM	1–2m	warm-up set
	3x3 @75% 1RM	2m between sets	
Snatch-Grip Conventional Deadlift, page 142	3x5	2m between sets	go heavy

CONDITIONING
do the following exercises as a circuit 4 times

Exercise	Set/Rep/Duration	Rest	Comments
Super Plank, page 156	30s	15s	
Goblet Squat, page 146	30s	15s	
Inverted Row, page 155	30s	15s	

PHASE III: Week 3, Day 1

WARM-UP

Exercise	Set/Rep/Duration	Rest	Comments
Foam roller			see "Incorporating Self-Myofascial Release" guidelines, page 39
Fixes			see "Are You Ready to Olympic Lift?" on page 28 for the self-assessment fixes you should do
Fast Feet Drill, page 161	3x10s	5s	
Side Shuffle, page 164	2x10s:10s	10s	
Bootstrapper, page 154	1x45s		

MAIN WORKOUT

Exercise	Set/Rep/Duration	Rest	Comments
Clean, page 104	1x3 @60% 1RM	1–2m	warm-up set
	1x3 @70% 1RM	1–2m	warm-up set
	3x3 @85% 1RM	2m between sets	
Barbell Front Squat, page 145	3x3	2m between sets	go heavy
Press, page 109	3x3	2m between sets	go heavy

CONDITIONING
do the following exercises as a circuit 3 times

Exercise	Set/Rep/Duration	Rest	Comments
Double Kettlebell Front Squat, page 147	30s	60s	go heavier than last week; you have longer rest periods
Burpee, page 161	30s	60s	
Side Plank, page 157	30s:30s	60s	

PHASE III: Week 3, Day 2

WARM-UP

Exercise	Set/Rep/Duration	Rest	Comments
Foam roller			see "Incorporating Self-Myofascial Release" guidelines, page 39
Fixes			see "Are You Ready to Olympic Lift?" on page 28 for the self-assessment fixes you should do
Kettlebell Turkish Get-Up, page 158	1x3 r/l		
Box Jump, page 149	1x10		
Carioca, page 160	2x15s:15s	15s	

MAIN WORKOUT

Exercise	Set/Rep/Duration	Rest	Comments
Snatch, page 138	1x3 @60% 1RM	1–2m	warm-up set
	1x3 @70% 1RM	1–2m	warm-up set
	3x3 @85% 1RM		
Overhead Squat, page 119	3x3	2m between sets	go heavy
Push Press, page 111	3x3	2m between sets	go heavy

CONDITIONING
do the following exercises as a circuit 3 times

Exercise	Set/Rep/Duration	Rest	Comments
Double Kettlebell Dead Snatch, page 148	30s	60s	go heavier than last week; you have longer rest periods
Mountain Climber, page 162	30s	60s	
Alternating Waves, page 166	30s	60s	

PHASE III: Week 3, Day 3

WARM-UP

Exercise	Set/Rep/Duration	Rest	Comments
Foam roller			see "Incorporating Self-Myofascial Release" guidelines, page 39
Fixes			see "Are You Ready to Olympic Lift?" on page 28 for the self-assessment fixes you should do
Bear Crawl, page 162 / Spiderman Crawl, page 163	1x30s	30s	do most advanced variation you can with good form
Half Get-Up, page 158	1x3 r/l		perform Turkish Get-Up until seated position, then return to the floor
Split Squat/Lunge variation, page 150	1x30s:30s	30s	do most advanced variation (Split Squat, Forward Lunge, Reverse Lunge, or Jumping Lunge) you can with good form

MAIN WORKOUT

Exercise	Set/Rep/Duration	Rest	Comments
Clean & Jerk	1x5 @60% 1RM		this is a combination of the Full Clean from the Floor (page 104) followed by the Split Jerk (page 115); warm-up set
	1x3 @70% 1RM		warm-up set
	3x3 @85% 1RM		
Snatch-Grip Conventional Deadlift, page 142	3x3	2m between sets	go heavy

CONDITIONING
do the following exercises as a circuit 3 times

Exercise	Set/Rep/Duration	Rest	Comments
Super Plank, page 156	30s	60s	
Goblet Squat, page 146	30s	60s	go heavier than last week; you have longer rest periods
Inverted Row, page 155	30s	60s	

PHASE III: Week 4, Day 1

WARM-UP

Exercise	Set/Rep/Duration	Rest	Comments
Foam roller			see "Incorporating Self-Myofascial Release" guidelines, page 39
Fixes			see "Are You Ready to Olympic Lift?" on page 28 for the self-assessment fixes you should do
Fast Feet Drill, page 161	3x10s	5s	
Side Shuffle, page 164	3x10s:10s	10s	
Bootstrapper, page 154	1x45s		

MAIN WORKOUT

Exercise	Set/Rep/Duration	Rest	Comments
Clean, page 104	1x3 @60% 1RM		
	1x3 @70% 1RM		
	5x1 @90% 1RM		5 singles; rest in between each rep
Barbell Front Squat, page 145	3x3		
Press, page 109	3x3		

CONDITIONING
do the following exercises as a circuit 3 times

Exercise	Set/Rep/Duration	Rest	Comments
Double Kettlebell Front Squat, page 147	30s	15s	
Burpee, page 161	30s	15s	
Side Plank, page 157	30s:30s	60s	

PHASE III: Week 4, Day 2

WARM-UP

Exercise	Set/Rep/Duration	Rest	Comments
Foam roller			see "Incorporating Self-Myofascial Release" guidelines, page 39
Fixes			see "Are You Ready to Olympic Lift?" on page 28 for the self-assessment fixes you should do
Kettlebell Turkish Get-Up, page 158	1x5 r/l		
Box Jump, page 149	1x12		
Carioca, page 160	3x15s:15s	15s	

MAIN WORKOUT

Exercise	Set/Rep/Duration	Rest	Comments
Snatch, page 138	1x3 @60% 1RM		
	1x3 @70% 1RM		
	5x1 @90% 1RM		5 singles; rest in between each rep
Overhead Squat, page 119	3x3		
Push Press, page 111	3x3		

CONDITIONING
do the following exercises as a circuit 4 times

Exercise	Set/Rep/Duration	Rest	Comments
Double Kettlebell Dead Snatch, page 148	30s	15s	
Mountain Climber, page 162	30s	15s	
Alternating Waves, page 166	30s	60s	

WARM-UP

Exercise	Set/Rep/Duration	Rest	Comments
Foam roller			see "Incorporating Self-Myofascial Release" guidelines, page 39
Fixes			see "Are You Ready to Olympic Lift?" on page 28 for the self-assessment fixes you should do
Bear Crawl, page 162 / Spiderman Crawl, page 163	2x30s	30s	do most advanced variation you can with good form
Half Get-Up, page 158	1x5 r/l		perform Turkish Get-Up until seated position, then return to the floor
Split Squat/Lunge variation, page 150	2x30s:30s	30s	do most advanced variation (Split Squat, Forward Lunge, Reverse Lunge, or Jumping Lunge) you can with good form

MAIN WORKOUT

Exercise	Set/Rep/Duration	Rest	Comments
Clean & Jerk	1x3 @60% 1RM		this is a combination of the Full Clean from the Floor (page 104) followed by the Split Jerk (page 115)
	1x3 @70% 1RM		
	5x1 @90% 1RM		5 singles; rest in between each rep
Snatch-Grip Conventional Deadlift, page 142	3x3		

CONDITIONING
do the following exercises as a circuit 4 times

Exercise	Set/Rep/Duration	Rest	Comments
Super Plank, page 156	30s	15s	
Goblet Squat, page 146	30s	15s	
Inverted Row, page 155	30s	15s	

Now that you've completed Phase III, you should be a pretty good Olympic lifter. You might not win any competitions yet, but you should be able to hold your own if you choose to compete.

You can repeat any of these phases using the appropriate weight at any time. In Phase I, you'd use lighter weights instead of PVC or an unweighted bar but it will help you to revisit the basics and hone your technique.

PART 3
THE LIFTS

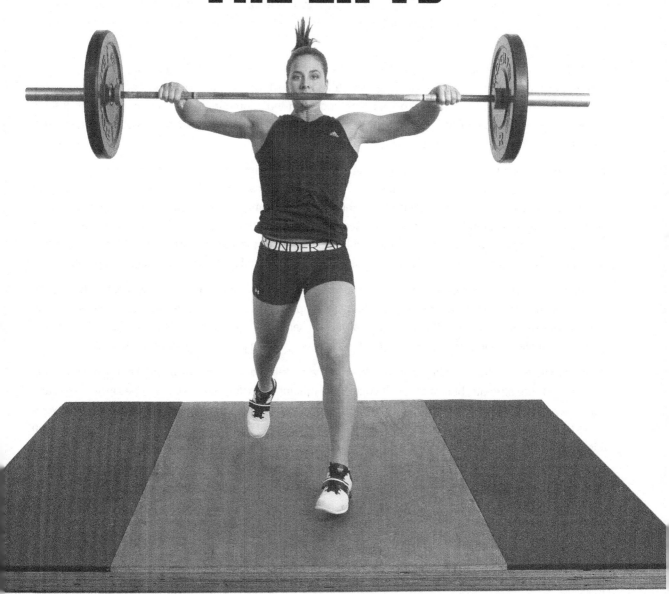

THE CLEAN

The clean by itself is not part of Olympic competition—the clean and jerk is. So why dedicate so much time on just the clean? Because it's the toughest and most technical part of the lift. In addition, it can make you very strong and powerful without doing the jerk. Also, if you have shoulder issues, doing the jerk may be contra-indicated.

The full clean is a very powerful, explosive movement that requires the use of your entire body to execute properly, especially with a heavy load. Even with a lighter load, when you use proper technique, you work almost every muscle in the body. Take your time and learn the segments before attempting to do the full movement. Remember, quality of movement is more important than how many reps you do or how much weight you lift. Ignoring this point is asking for an injury.

The clean incorporates a pull from the floor and a front squat with explosive power from your hips, which is transferred through your core to pull the bar off the floor and caught or racked across the fronts of your shoulders (the anterior deltoids). The power in this lift comes from your lower body: the momentum of your hips is what lifts the weight, while your arms and hands hold the bar steady. As the bar approaches chest level, there's a quick elbow reversal and you pull yourself under the bar, dropping into a deep squat while catching the bar across your shoulders. You finish the clean by standing up with your knees straight.

The clean is a technical movement, and there are several places where things can go wrong. For this reason I break the movement into learnable chunks that can be practiced as standalone exercises. This allows you to focus on specific sections of the lifts, especially if one segment is problematic. Once you can do each part proficiently (notice I didn't say mastered—that takes years), you can put them together for the full movement.

Some people may not be able to do a full clean into a rock-bottom squat. For many, it's a question of hip mobility and core strength, but for others it could be a structural problem, such as the bones in your hips and pelvis won't allow you to go all the way into a deep squat. If it's a bone issue, sorry, all the training in the world won't fix the problem. If it's a muscular imbalance, you're in luck. I've included a number of exercise fixes in this book to help you improve hip mobilization (see "Squat & Shoulder Mobility Assessment" on page 29 to see if you're ready for the lifts or if you require further work).

Here's the progression for learning the clean:

Scarecrow Clean (page 91)

High Pull (page 89)

TERMINOLOGY

FIRST PULL. The first pull from the floor looks like a deadlift but isn't: Your knees move back, your torso and hips rise together until the bar passes your knees, then your hips move forward and your torso comes up. If the first pull doesn't go well, the clean won't go well. In fact, doing the first pull from the floor is where most people, including professional weightlifters, have problems.

HANG POSITION. The hang position (see the hang position description on page 26) is useful in training movement segments, helping those who have difficulty with the first pull. Doing the clean variations from the hang position still requires a lot of power generation, but it's less technically difficult than pulling from the floor. Typically you'll use boxes, blocks, or a squat rack to get the bar up to the proper height.

RACK POSITION. The rack position (see the rack position description on page 26) can be very uncomfortable as it requires a lot of mobility in the wrists and fingers as well as forearm flexibility. Mobility in the upper back (thoracic spine) is also necessary to achieve a good rack position.

HIGH PULL. To perform the high pull, drive your heels down and hips forward from the hang position. That will bring your torso up and cause the bar to rise rapidly. Your arms, mostly through momentum, come up until your elbows are higher than your shoulders and the bar is about chest level. Some people may come up on the balls of their feet—that's normal. The high pull can be further broken down based on where you start it: below the knees, just above the knees, or mid-thigh. The farther down the bar starts, the longer range of motion and therefore the more power generation. Starting at mid-thigh is tougher because it's harder to generate as much force due to the shorter range of motion.

HANG CLEAN. This movement starts from the hang position and ends with the bar racked while dropping into a full squat.

POWER CLEAN. The power clean is caught with a high-squat position rather than your thighs parallel to your hips or deeper; the starting point is either from the floor or from the hang position.

FULL CLEAN. Started from the floor, this is caught in rack position as you drop under the bar into a full rock-bottom squat.

GRIP. The most straightforward position is a conventional *clean-width overhand grip:* Your palms face backward while your thumbs are around the bar and on top of your fingers. You can also use a clean-width hook grip, where your thumbs are also around the bar but under your fingers. The *hook grip* puts your thumb in a more advantageous position, making it stronger than the conventional version. It does take a while to get used to, though. To use the hook grip, place the web of your thumbs on the bar so that your palms face backward, then wrap your fingers around the thumb and bar.

HAND PLACEMENT. If your hands aren't in the proper place at the beginning of the lift, it will be difficult and painful to hold the bar in rack position. Here's how to check if your hands are in the correct place.

Hook grip: Standing with an unweighted bar, your arms are straight and your hands hang about mid-thigh, palms facing backward.

Overhand grip: Place your hands far enough apart so that you just brush the sides of your thighs with your thumbs.

PULLING STANCE (STARTING FOOT POSITION). Place your feet hip-width apart, not any wider, and turned out slightly.

SQUAT STANCE (ENDING FOOT POSITION). Your ending foot stance depends on your hip mobility and squat depth. For power cleans, where you're in a partial squat, your feet will only go a little wider than your pulling stance. If you're doing rock-bottom squats, your stance will be a little more than shoulder-width apart.

DETERMINING YOUR SQUAT STANCE

Your squat stance will differ depending on whether you're doing a high squat or a full-depth squat. You should also play around a little and do some full-depth squats to find your optimal squat-stance foot.

1. Stand with an unweighted bar in rack position, your feet shoulder-width apart and toes turned out slightly.

2. Squat down as far as you can while keeping your knees over your toes and your upper body as upright as possible. Note the depth and how the position feels.

3. Return to standing by driving through your heels. Your torso comes up with your hips.

If the squat was deep (thighs below parallel) and it felt comfortable, you've found your squat stance. If not, move your feet a little wider and repeat until you find the stance that's right for you.

Note: At this point, you may never find a good stance. If that's the case, you need to work on your hip and upper back mobility and core stability. Since most people don't really need to go rock bottom, don't worry about it for now: Practice the deep squat as an assistance exercise. Later you can work on it as part of the clean.

DISSECTING THE MOVEMENT

Before you attempt the full clean movement, I've dissected the key parts of the lift. I highly recommend starting your practice with a 5- or 6-foot piece of ¾-inch-diameter PVC and progressing to an unweighted barbell. As you get the movements down, you can start to *slowly* add weight to the bar. When practicing the first pull with a bar, use light bumper plates so that the bar will always be at the correct height.

SHRUGGING & COMING UP ON THE BALLS OF THE FEET

If you watch good Olympic lifters, you'll see them come up on the balls of their feet as the bar comes up toward rack position. You may also notice what appears to be a shrug. During training, especially with beginners, coming up on the balls of the feet is taught to help generate power and supposedly to get the bar higher. However, what's really happening is the transition of the feet from the pulling position to the squatting position. Coming up on the balls of the feet is momentary and is a result of the power being put into the bar; it shouldn't be deliberate. Training to come up on the balls of the feet will slow you down since you're thinking about it. It should just happen naturally.

The same is true for the "shrug," which occurs during the second pull (high pull) part of the clean. Beginners are coached a little, but if the clean is done correctly, the shoulders will naturally rise without thought or effort. They rise due to momentum and relaxed arms and shoulders. It's not a deliberate shrug.

Hang Position

The hang position allows you to start from an easier position than the floor in order to learn the various segments of the clean. Since the first pull is pretty technical, starting from the hang allows you to practice other pieces of the clean without dealing with the first pull. If you're a beginner to lifting and using PVC or an unweighted bar, just pick it up. Otherwise, follow these instructions:

1. Place a bar with light bumper or training plates on jerk blocks so that the bar is about knee level. Stand in front of the bar so that it's above the middle portion of your feet.

2. Bend your knees and grab the bar in a hook grip, elbows straight. Your hands are far enough apart so that you just brush the sides of your thighs with your thumbs.

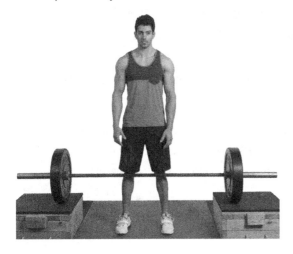

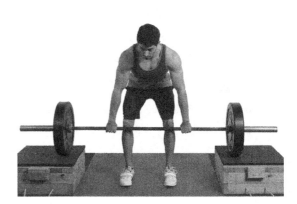

3. Come up so that the bar is above your knees but don't stand up all the way. At this point your hips are back, your knees are slightly bent, and your torso is inclined to about 45 degrees above parallel. The exact angle depends on your build. If your torso is bent over too far, you'll wind up using your back too much. If your torso is too upright, you won't be able to generate enough power.

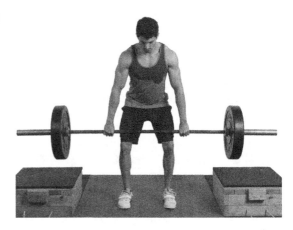

Muscle High Pull

The high pull with a PVC is merely a training exercise to get you used to the movement of the body and bar. In this training move, you're actually using your muscles to lift the PVC pipe into position. When doing the actual high pull at speed, momentum lifts the bar, not the arm muscles. To begin, move slowly and only use your arms until you learn the positions. Note that all beginners should do this with a PVC pipe; you'll get to the unweighted bar soon enough.

1. Start from the hang position.

2. As you push your hips forward and your torso comes up, raise your elbows up as high as possible to lift the bar up to about chest level.

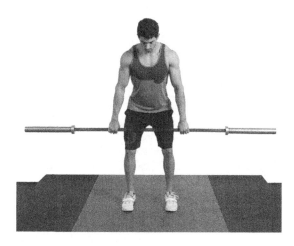

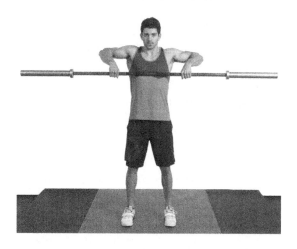

3. Reverse the movement by lowering your arms and pushing your hips back until you return to hang position.

You may find the high pull position uncomfortable at the top. This is likely due to shoulder and upper back mobility issues, which need to be addressed quickly to prevent injury. If you experience shoulder pain during the high pull, you need to see a physical therapist and get checked out for a possible impingement.

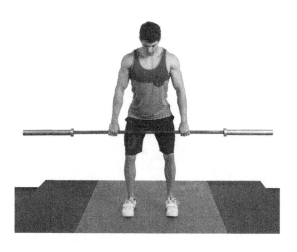

If you just feel tight and uncomfortable, you need to work on opening your shoulders and upper back. You don't need to perform the exercises in the order below. Try them all then pick the three or four that give you the most trouble. These are the ones you need to practice several times a day, if possible, and definitely before you start to lift.

1. Shoulder Dislocate (page 172)

2. Half-Kneeling Halo (page 171) and Tall-Kneeling Halo (page 171)

3. Band-Assisted Pec Stretch (page 171)

4. Quad Extension Rotation (page 170)

5. Side-Lying Windmill (page 172)

6. Bretzel (page 173)

7. Lat Stretch with Band (page 173)

8. Arm Bar (page 173)

High Pull

Once you feel comfortable with the high pull from hang position using the PVC, it's time to advance to an unweighted bar and add some speed to it. This portion of the clean is referred to as the second pull when the clean is done from the floor.

1. Start from hang position with an unweighted bar.

2. Drive your hips forward explosively. Your knees straighten and your torso comes up.

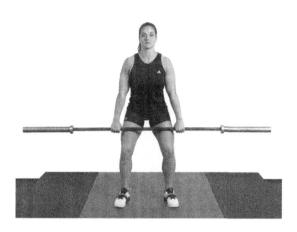
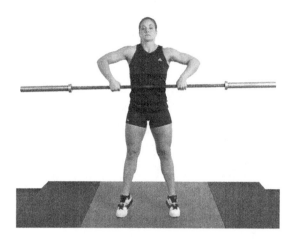

3. As the bar rises from momentum, bend your elbows to the sides, allowing the bar to rise to about chest level.

4. To return to hang position, let the bar drop down, pushing your hips back and allowing your knees to bend a little to absorb the energy of the bar.

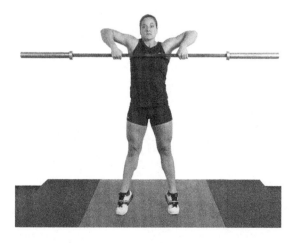
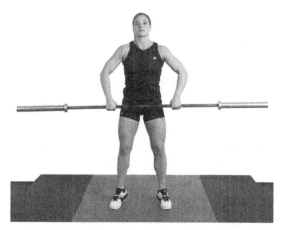

Don't hold the high pull—just get it up and back down with control. The bar should feel like it's floating up; there should be no excess tension in your arms, shoulders, or hands. If you find yourself rising up on your toes or your shoulders are going up too, that's okay—it's a natural function of the movement, but don't force it to happen.

Scarecrow Clean

Initially you should use your PVC to practice getting the bar racked from the high pull. Once you're comfortable, you can switch to an unweighted bar.

1. Hold a bar at chest level in a hook grip.

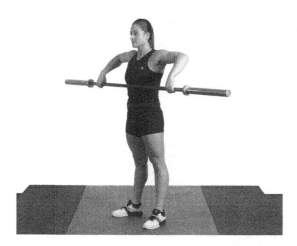

2. Quickly rotate your elbows down, under, and up until they point forward with your upper arms parallel to the floor. Your hands should naturally open up and your thumb should come out. The bar should be across the fronts of your shoulders, resting on the fingertips and lightly touching your throat. Try to create a shelf. The bar should not be out on your biceps. This is called "rack position."

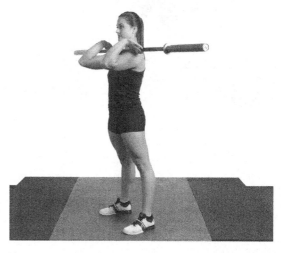

If you're very tight in the forearms, wrists, shoulders, or lats, you may find that you can't get the bar on your shoulders. That's okay for now—keep working on your elbow rotation with the PVC. When you feel you can do it properly, go to an unweighted bar.

Once you move to an unweighted bar, it should cause enough of a stretch in your fingers, wrists, and forearms so that the bar does end up on the shoulders. This may feel quite uncomfortable until you gain some flexibility in those tight areas. The best thing to do is keep practicing the rack from the high pull; over time you'll be able to hold the rack without any issues.

Muscle Clean

This is a drill to learn how to get the bar up and into rack position without dealing with your legs. Use a PVC or unweighted bar.

1. Stand tall holding an unweighted bar in a hook grip. The bar should be touching your thighs.

2. Without using your legs, pull the bar up until it reaches your upper chest. Your elbows should be up and out just like when doing the high pull.

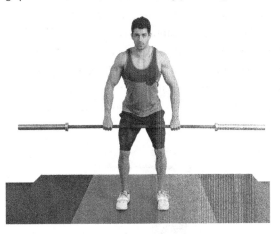

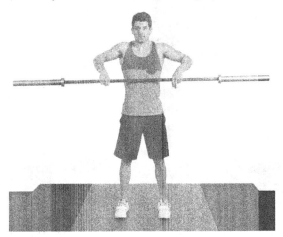

3. Drop your elbows and rotate them forward and up so that they point straight ahead. As your elbows rotate, release your grip. The bar should rest on the fronts of your shoulders and your fingertips should be holding the bar in place.

Remember, this is a just a drill.

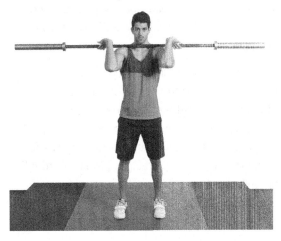

Getting under the Bar

Getting under the bar is another forceful pull, sometimes called the third pull. As the bar reaches it's highest level and your feet begin transitioning to the squat stance, you use the bar to pull against in order to get below it. This happens at the same time your elbows are turning over. This helps you to get under faster, but can be tough to get the hang of.

The bar is the pivot point—you (as opposed to your elbows or shoulders) are trying to rotate around and under it. If you rotate around your elbows, the bar will travel away from you, making it much more difficult to rack.

Foot Transition

Doing the clean properly, especially with a heavy load, requires (and develops) very fast feet. The ability to quickly shift your feet from the initial hip-width stance to squat stance is essential. If your feet are slow, your timing will be off and getting into a full squat will be tough.

Your feet are about hip-width apart during the pulling phase, but when you go into rack, especially with a full squat, your squat stance's foot position must be slightly wider than the typical shoulder-width distance. The exact position varies from person to person and depends on hip, ankle, and upper back mobility.

For now, we'll focus on the partial squat and leave the discussion on full-depth squats and mobility for later.

Drop Squat

This is a very fast movement and is like you're falling into the squat as opposed to jumping into it. The faster you can move your feet, the more successful you'll be with both the clean and the snatch.

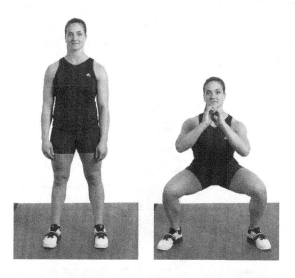

1. Place your feet in the pulling position with your arms by your sides.

2. Now quickly drive your feet out and land in a partial squat with your hips just a little above parallel. Try to keep your feet as close to the floor as possible; don't come up on the balls of your feet.

Practice the foot movement for 10 reps. When you feel comfortable with the footwork, rack an unweighted bar and try again and see if anything changes. A little deviation is okay, but if you're going a lot wider with the bar than without, you need to adjust your foot movement with the unweighted bar so that it's the same as without a bar. This is just for practice. The actual foot movement happens as the bar transitions from high pull to rack.

Now we'll drill the foot transition at speed. It's normal for your feet to make a lot of noise when landing. However, many people try to artificially stomp the floor to make the noise, which misses the point. If you try to force the stomping, you slow yourself down.

1. Start from scarecrow (high pull) position with a PVC pipe.

2. Quickly explode your feet out to the squat position and simultaneously start to move the bar into rack position.

3. Land flat on the floor in a partial squat; the bar should be in rack.

4. Stand up and return to scarecrow position and repeat.

Once you have that down, repeat the drill with an unweighted bar.

Now it's time to put together some of the pieces into a fluid movement.

Hang Power Clean

This is a very fast movement that requires coordination, timing, and attention to form. There are many places where things can go wrong and it's wise to take your time and practice the segments. When beginners add weight to the bar, it tends to change their technique, so start with an unweighted bar and practice until things feel good. When you're ready to add weight, start again with working on individual segments. Video yourself to double-check your form. Once you have it down, add 5 pounds to the bar and begin the process once again. If you find problem areas, practice that segment with the extra weight. You may find yourself naturally coming up on the balls of your feet as the bar reaches its apex. This allows a slightly faster foot transition and a little more power in the second pull, but if you stay up on the balls you'll actually move slower.

1. Start from hang position with an unweighted bar.

2. Explode your hips forward; as your torso comes up, the bar should float up. As the bar rises from momentum, allow your elbows to bend and point out to the sides, allowing the bar to rise to about chest level.

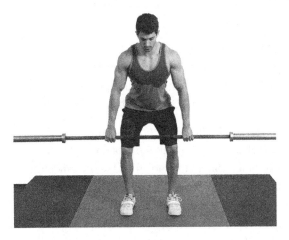

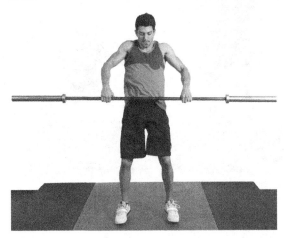

3. When the bar reaches chest level, quickly move your feet to the squat stance and pull yourself under the bar into a partial squat. At the same time, quickly rotate your elbows down, under, and up until they point forward with the upper arms parallel to the floor. Catch the bar in rack as your heels come down on the floor shoulder-width apart. Your hips should be back, your knees partially bent, and your torso upright. Bending your legs allows them to absorb the weight of the bar as you catch it in rack instead of your shoulders and arms taking the load.

4. Once in rack position, stand up.

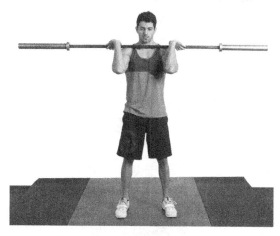

Drop the bar back to hang position.

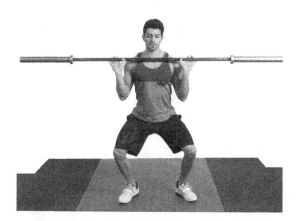

Hang Clean

When you're proficient in the hang power clean, it's time to move to the hang clean. Remember: You must practice, practice, practice. Don't rush the steps; learn the movements and master them.

1. Start from hang position with an unweighted bar.

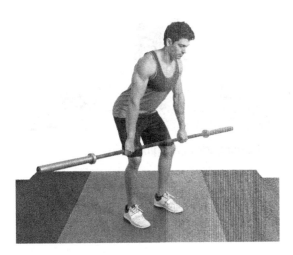

2. Drive your hips forward explosively; as your torso comes up, the bar should float up. As the bar rises from momentum, bend your elbows to the sides, allowing the bar to rise to about chest level. Allow your elbows to bend as they did during the High Pull (page 89).

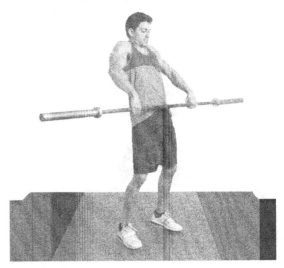

3. When the bar reaches chest level, quickly move your feet to the squat stance and pull yourself under the bar into a full squat. At the same time, quickly rotate your elbows down, under, and up until they point forward with the upper arms parallel to the floor. Catch the bar in rack as your heels come down on the floor shoulder-width apart. Your hips should be back, your knees partially bent, and your torso upright. Bending your legs allows them to absorb the weight of the bar as you catch it in rack instead of your shoulders and arms taking the load.

4. Once in rack position, stand up.

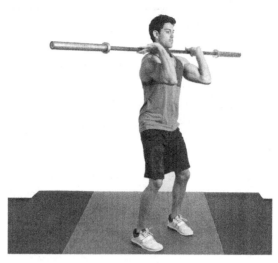

Drop the bar back to hang position.

First Pull

The first pull from the floor tends to be the trickiest part of the clean and the snatch—even seasoned Olympic lifters can have difficulty with this part. To practice, work on the first pull, initially starting with an unweighted barbell. You'll need to use blocks to raise the bar up to the same height it would be with plates. As you become used to the movement, add light to moderate weight. Use light bumper or training plates so that the bar is always at the same height from the floor. Don't pull too fast or it will slow down the second pull. A moderate and deliberate speed is best.

Set-Up

1. Place the bar on the floor using light bumper or training plates to elevate the bar to the normal height. The bar should be over the base of your big toes.

2. Place your hands on your thighs and push your hips back until your hands reach your knees.

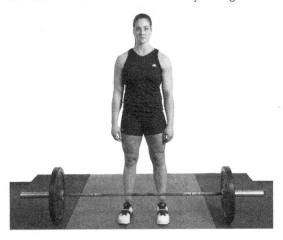

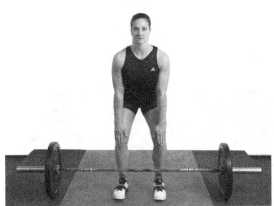

3. Sit your hips straight down. Your shins should be forward slightly and arms vertical. Grab the bar in a hook grip. Your hand placement on the bar is exactly where it was when holding the PVC pipe or bar while standing.

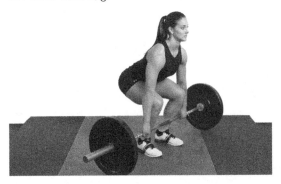

Pull

1. From the set-up position, drive your feet into the floor.

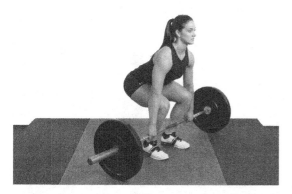

2. Move your knees back as your hips come up so that the bar doesn't go around your knees. As the bar passes your knees, drive your hips forward explosively and lift your torso.

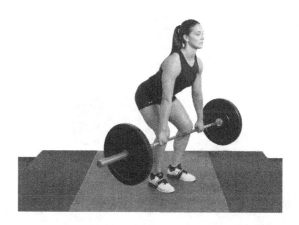

3. Finish the first pull by standing tall. The bar should be about mid-thigh. Normally you wouldn't finish by standing, but at this beginning stage our goal is to get the bar off the floor successfully.

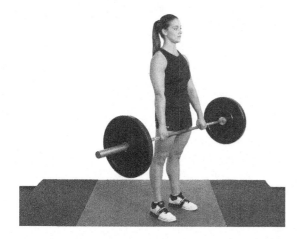

Returning the Bar to the Floor

1. Push your hips back, keeping the bar slightly off your thighs. Your torso will lean forward, moving with your hips. Your knees remain straight but "soft" until the bar goes below them.

2. With control, bend your knees more and lower your hips until the bar is resting on the floor. Keep your lats tight and abs braced while lowering the bar. Don't drop the bar, especially at this stage.

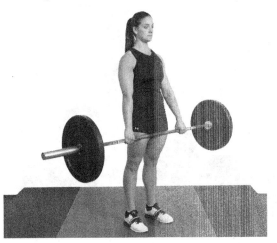

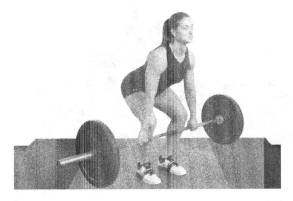

The bar path is vertical during this first pull as well as when lowering it to the floor. If the bar swings out around your knees, you'll lose power because the center of mass between the bar and your body shifts forward. The bar may slightly brush your shins, but only slightly. The bar should not rip your shins—this is not acceptable technique. If this does happen, your shoulders may be too far back or you aren't getting your knees back soon enough.

Clean-Grip Halting Deadlift

As you get used to the first pull, you can move a little faster and use a little more weight, but don't go heavy until you have the technique down pat.

1. Pull from the floor to 1 inch off the floor, pause for 2–3 seconds, then lower the bar to the floor with control.

2. Reset and pull to 1 inch off the floor, pause 2–3 seconds, then pull to just below your knees. Pause for 2–3 seconds then lower it with control to the floor.

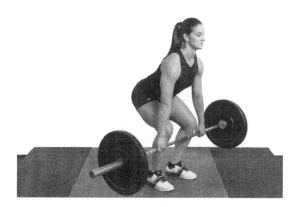
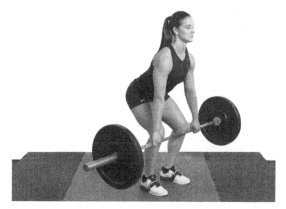

3. Reset. Pull to 1 inch off the floor, pause for 2–3 seconds, then pull to just below your knees. Pause for 2–3 seconds, pull to just above your knees, pause for 2–3 seconds, then lower it to the floor with control.

4. Reset and do step 3 again but, instead of lowering it after you get just above your knees, bring it up to mid-thigh and pause for 2–3 seconds before lowering it to the floor with control.

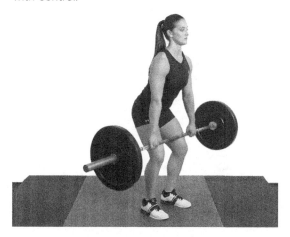
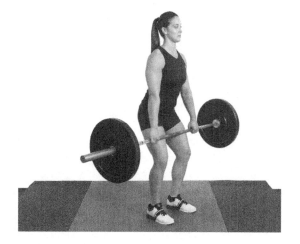

Do that 5 times and you'll get a lot stronger throughout the phases of the first pull and deadlifts in general. If it's pretty easy, add a little weight and repeat.

Once you have that down, do the full first pull to mid-thigh without stopping. Drive through your hips and push your feet into the floor. The speed of the bar is slow during the first pull compared to the rest of the lift. If you move too fast here, it will actually slow down your second pull.

Power Clean from the Floor

Initiate the first pull as described above and, as the bar reaches mid-thigh, explode—really snap your hips forward and your torso up. The bar should brush your mid-thigh but don't let it bounce off or it will travel away from you and you'll probably miss the lift. Use your lats to keep the bar close to your body.

The bar should be traveling up just as it did with the high pull with your elbows up. As the bar reaches chest level, quickly get under the bar into a partial squat (power clean). Finish by standing up.

1. Do the first pull to just above your knee with moderate speed.

2. Drive your hips forward explosively to initiate the second pull. The top of your head rises to the ceiling as you straighten your knees and extend your feet.

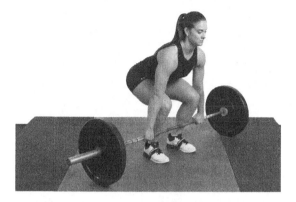

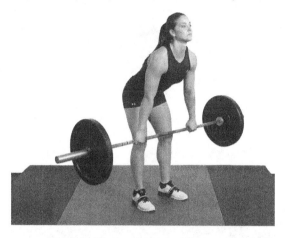

3. As the bar reaches chest level, quickly drive your feet out to the squat position, reversing your elbows and getting under the bar.

4. Catch the bar in rack as your feet plant and your knees bend into a partial squat.

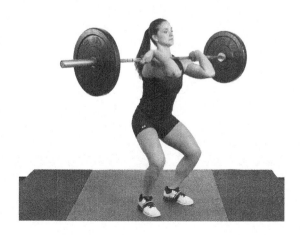

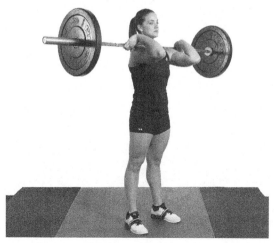

5. Once in rack position, stand up.

Full Clean

All that's left now is getting into the rock-bottom squat. Let's begin by racking a bar and doing some front squats to check your squat depth and mechanics. Your mobility, shin and thigh bone length, as well as your torso and arm length, all play a part in your exact position. This squat stance should look the same regardless of where the load is on your body—in rack, on your back, using bodyweight, or with a kettlebell. *Note:* If you can't get your thighs below parallel or keep your torso close to vertical when doing the squat, you should not do cleans into a full squat.

1. Stand with an unweighted bar in rack position with your feet shoulder-width apart and toes turned out slightly.

2. Move your feet to squat stance. Keeping your elbows up, squat down. Your torso should stay as vertical as possible while your knees track with your toes and are angled forward somewhat but not in front of your toes.

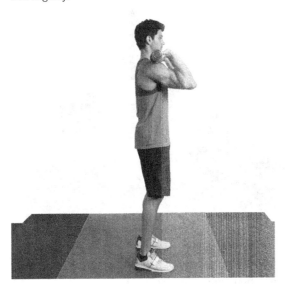

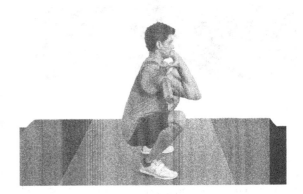

If you can do a deep squat, you're ready to put it all together.

1. Place the bar on the floor using training plates or light bumpers. The bar should be over the base of your big toes.

2. Place your hands on your thighs and push your hips back until your hands reach your knees.

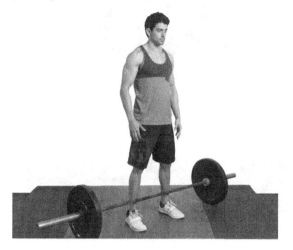
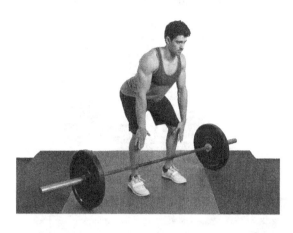

3. Sit your hips straight down. Your shins should be forward slightly and arms vertical. Grab the bar in a hook grip.

4. From the set-up position, drive your feet into the floor. Move your knees back as your hips come up so the bar doesn't go around the knees.

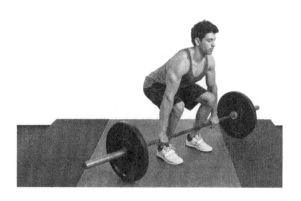
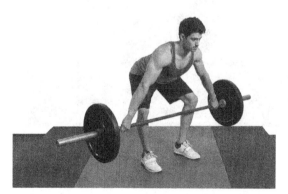

5. As the bar passes your knees, drive your hips forward explosively and lift your torso to start the second pull. The top of your head rises to the ceiling as you straighten your knees and extend your feet. Let the bar rise up, guiding it with your arms.

6. As the bar reaches chest level, reverse your elbows and at the same time drive your feet to squat stance.

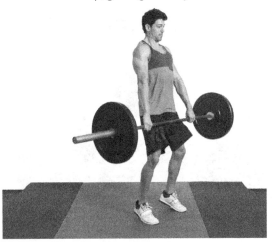

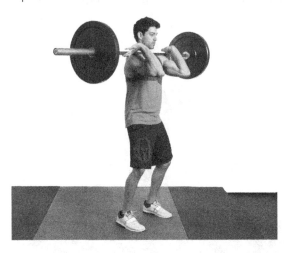

7. Catch the bar in rack position as your feet plant and drop into a full-depth squat.

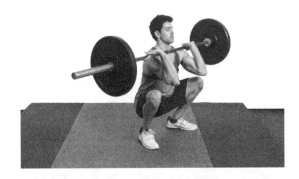

THE JERK

To perform the jerk without the clean, you'll need to utilize blocks or a squat rack. For beginners, this is the way to practice before integrating the full clean and jerk. As you get better, you can add in the clean.

The idea behind the jerk, regardless of stance or position of the bar, is that you're trying to get under the bar as quickly as possible. Don't try to push the bar up—you want to go down while the bar remains fairly stationary. Think about standing on a chair in a doorway with your palms up on the top part of the doorframe. You want to straighten your elbows. How are you going to do that? The doorframe isn't going to move no matter how hard you push it. The only option is to push your hips back and bend your knees, which allows your elbows to straighten.

There are several practice exercises used for learning the jerk:

Press from Behind the Neck (page 108)

Push Press (page 111) and a Push Press from Behind the Neck (page 110)

Power Jerk in Front of the Neck (page 114) / Power Jerk from Behind the Neck (page 113)

Split Jerk (page 115) / Split Jerk Behind the Neck (page 115)

Doing the practice variations from behind the neck helps shoulder mobility and teaches a vertical bar path. When the bar is overhead, it should be directly above the base of the neck regardless of whether the movement started in front of or behind the neck. When the bar is in front, in rack position, it's a little tougher to keep it vertical; the behind-the-neck variations reinforce the end point.

TERMINOLOGY

Just as with the clean, there are two foot placements: the drive stance and the catch stance.

DRIVE STANCE. The feet are a little wider than hip width and turned out slightly.

CATCH STANCE. This position varies depending on whether you're catching with parallel feet or from a split position. The first option is a *parallel stance*, with the feet moving out to the sides a little. When you use this stance, you'll be receiving the bar overhead by dropping into a partial squat. Some people prefer the parallel stance, especially when using lighter weights. Also, for those who practice double kettlebell jerks, the parallel-stance barbell jerk is similar to the movement of the kettlebell jerk.

The second position is a *split stance*, where one foot moves forward and the other backward as you drop into a lunge stance under the bar. The split stance is much more stable and makes catching and holding the bar easier. It also allows you to get under the bar deeper and faster than the parallel stance.

HAND PLACEMENT. This is the same as the clean: Keeping your arms down and elbows straight, you should just be able to brush the sides of your thighs with your thumbs. When you stand up after catching the clean, it's okay to bounce the bar off your shoulders slightly to reposition your hands if necessary.

KNEE DIP. Both the push press and jerk use an initial knee dip to get the bar moving upward. In the push press your knees end up straight with the bar overhead. In the jerk, your feet either move to the wide catch stance or the split stance after your knees straighten. In both cases, the dip provides momentum to the bar.

1. From the drive stance, dip your knees forward then quickly straighten them out. This is fast and explosive and should feel as though you're throwing the bar up instead of pressing it.

PRESSES

As you did with the clean, you'll start with a PVC pipe and progress to an unloaded barbell. When practicing the jerk from the rack position, your elbows will be down. They're up only during the catch phase of the clean. Once you've returned to standing, your elbows need to point down. This is due to the mechanics of the jerk and keeping the bar tight and connected to your body for optimal power and vertical bar path.

Press from Behind the Neck

1. Stand in drive stance with an unweighted bar behind your neck, eyes looking forward.

2. Press the bar straight up until your elbows are locked out.

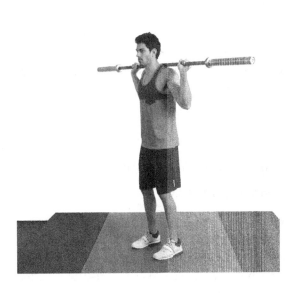

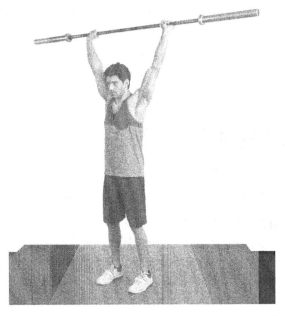

Get used to the overhead position, making sure the bar is over the base of your neck and the path is vertical.

Press

1. Stand in drive stance with an unweighted bar in rack position with your elbows pointing down instead of forward.

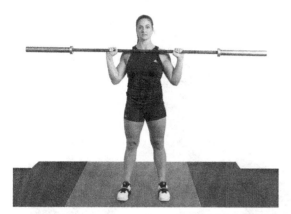

2. Press the bar straight up until your elbows are locked out while moving your head back so it's out of the way of the bar. Your knees don't bend throughout the movement. The bar should be over the base of your neck when your arms lock out. Your torso may lean forward slightly after the bar passes your head.

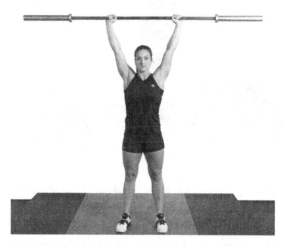

3. Lower the bar with control by bending your elbows until the bar touches the front of your deltoids (rack position with elbows down). To do another rep, press the bar back up. On your last rep, rotate your forearms behind and up. Allow your arms to straighten, bend your knees, and place the bar on the floor.

Push Press from Behind the Neck

1. Stand in drive stance with an unweighted bar behind your neck.

2. Dip your knees forward and down. Keep your feet flat on the floor.

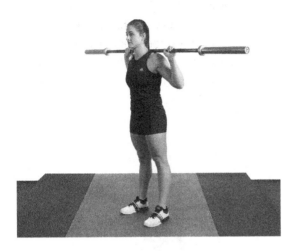

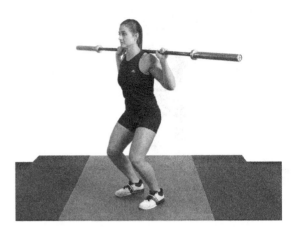

3. Quickly reverse the knee bend and drive the bar overhead as your knees straighten. The bar should be directly over the base of your neck where it started, with your elbows locked out and knees straight.

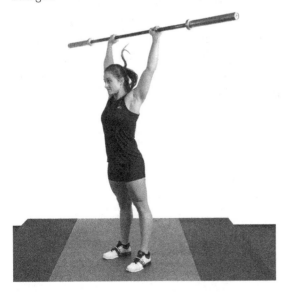

Push Press

1. Stand in drive stance with an unweighted bar in rack position, elbows pointing down instead of forward.

2. Drive your knees forward and down. Keep your feet flat on the floor.

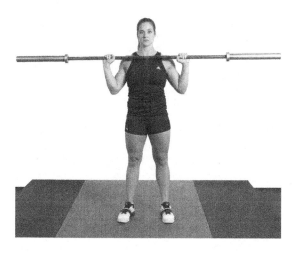

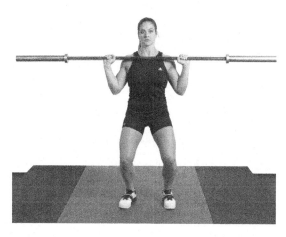

3. Quickly reverse the knee bend and drive the bar overhead as your knees straighten.

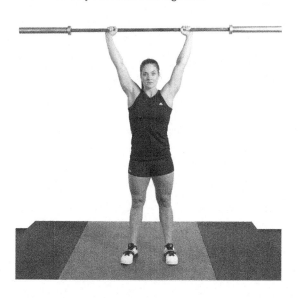

The bar should be over the base of your neck where it started, with your elbows locked and knees straight.

The jerk adds more legwork to the push press. Again, you're trying to get under the bar rather than move the bar up over you. In order to do that, use the knee dip to get your body, and therefore the bar, moving upward. By quickly shifting your feet and straightening your elbows, the bar will wind up overhead without pressing. If you catch the bar with bent elbows in either the parallel stance or the split stance, the lift won't count as a jerk because you would then have to press the bar out to lock your elbows.

GETTING INTO CATCH POSITION

The *parallel stance* is a quick outward movement of the feet similar to the way your feet move when catching a full clean. It's not a jump—your body is actually falling. How wide you go depends on your hip and shoulder mobility. If you have tighter shoulders, you'll probably have a wider stance. In fact, if you're very tight in the shoulders, you'll probably find that the split stance works better for you.

When you catch the jerk using the shoulder-width stance, you'll be dropping into a partial squat like in the hang and power cleans.

The *split stance* looks like a lunge—one foot is planted forward while the other is behind you.

- The rear foot and leg should be in line with or slightly outside the rear hip.
- The front foot and knee should be in line with the lead hip.
- The front shin is vertical with the front knee bent to about 20 degrees with respect to the floor.
- The rear knee is bent but not much. How much the knees bend will depend on how heavy the weight is. The heavier the load, the deeper the stance.
- The torso must remain vertical and the hips aligned under the shoulders.

Start with your feet in drive stance with your hands on your hips. Quickly drop to the split stance by moving one foot forward and the other back. Check your stance versus the description and pictures shown here. Remember, it's a drop, not a jump.

As you practice the drop, don't shift your torso front to back or to the sides. Your legs are the only things moving. You'll be trying to get under the bar and your torso must be stable to lock out your elbows and hold the bar.

Normally your dominant leg will go forward since it's stronger and that feels natural. Some people like to train the opposite side leg as well so they balance the workload on the legs. For beginner- to intermediate-level athletes, that's fine. However, if you're serious about competing, you should only train with your dominant leg forward.

JERKS

Power Jerk from Behind the Neck

1. Stand in drive stance with an unweighted bar behind your neck.

2. Drive your knees forward and down.

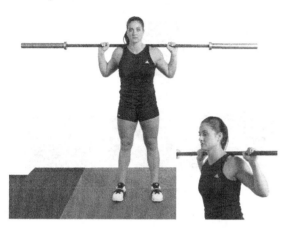

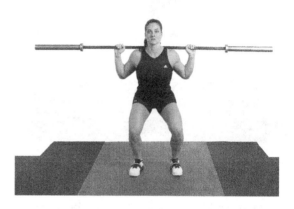

3. Explosively reverse the knee bend; as your knees straighten, quickly shift your feet wide. Your arms should be straightening as your feet land; your elbows should lock out as you drop into a partial squat.

4. Stand up, keeping your elbows locked out.

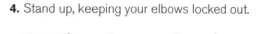

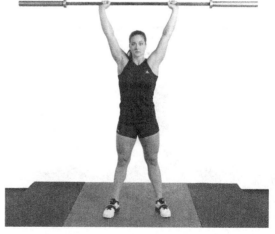

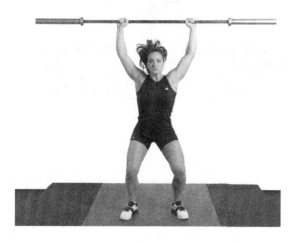

Power Jerk in Front of the Neck

1. Stand in drive stance with a bar in rack position, just as you did with the Push Press (page 111).

2. Drive your knees forward and down.

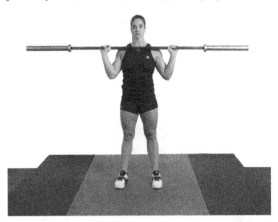

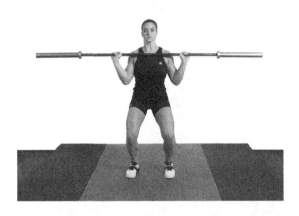

3. Explosively reverse the knee bend; as your knees straighten, quickly shift your feet wide. Your arms should be straightening as your feet land; your elbows should lock out as you drop into a partial squat.

4. Stand up, keeping your elbows locked out.

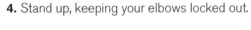

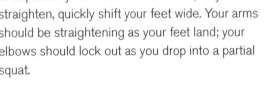

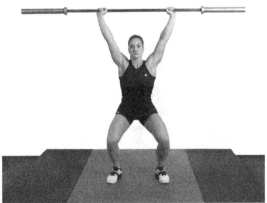

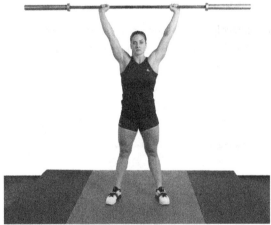

Split Jerk

When doing a split jerk, the initial set-up, knee dip, and drive are the same. The second phase is where the difference lies—your feet will move to a split stance instead of a squat position. The split stance is a bit faster and makes it easier for most athletes to get deeper under the bar than with the partial squat version.

You should've determined your dominant leg and foot position that's most comfortable for you while maintaining proper alignment (see page 112).

1. Stand in drive stance with a bar in rack position. Rack the bar as you did in the jerk in front of the neck.

2. Drive your knees forward and down.

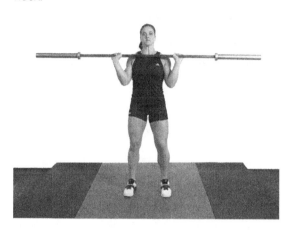

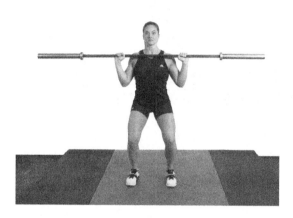

3. Explosively reverse the knee bend; as your knees straighten, quickly shift your feet into the split stance. At the same time, the bar should be rising overhead as your elbows straighten.

4. When your reach the split stance, your elbows should be locked out.

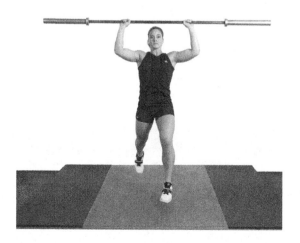

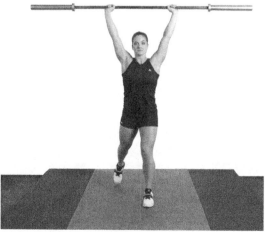

5. Return to standing by either bringing your back foot forward, your front foot back, or a little of both. Make sure your elbows stay locked.

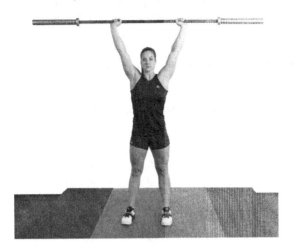

6. Lower the bar with control by bending your elbows until the bar reaches shoulder level. On your last rep, rotate your forearms so your elbows point up. Allow your arms to straighten, bend your knees, and place the bar on the floor.

When dropping into the split stance, your lead knee should already be bent to the proper depth. Don't land and then bend the knees more. The goal is to drop under as quickly as possible. When you land your feet and then bend your knees, the move is slower and may make you miss the lockout, especially with heavier weights.

You can also practice the split jerk with the jerk from behind the neck. Everything is the same except the start position of the bar.

SNATCHES

With the exception of the hand placement on the bar, the first portion of both the snatches and cleans are the same. However in the snatch, you must get under the bar faster and deeper because the bar is going directly overhead, not into rack position like in the clean. Getting the bar directly overhead requires more power and a lot more shoulder and hip mobility than the clean and jerk.

Consequently, you won't be able to snatch as much as you can clean. You also have a much more narrow margin of error when doing the snatch—being out of position or off with the timing even by just a fraction of a second can cause you to miss the lift. In the event of a miss, just let the bar travel in the direction it was going while you quickly move the other way. Don't try to rescue it.

TERMINOLOGY

SNATCH GRIP. The snatch grip is typically a very wide hook grip. To determine the hand placement on the bar:

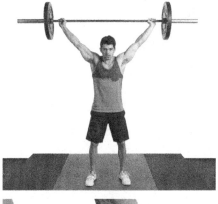

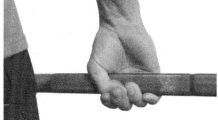

1. With a hook grip, hold a bar down in front of you, arms straight. Move your hands apart, which will bring the bar higher on your thighs until the bar is in the crease of your hips. You should be able to lift your knee up without the bar moving. Your elbows are straight throughout.

When the bar is overhead, your thumbs must come out, your wrists will be bent backward, and the bar will be across the center of your palms, which are facing up, not forward—you won't be able to hold a heavy bar with forward-facing palms.

FIRST PULL. The first pull for the snatch is the same as the first pull with the clean, the difference being the width of the hands on the bar, as described above

PULLING STANCE. The pulling stance is the same as the clean: Place your feet hip-width apart, not any wider, and turned out slightly (no more than 10 degrees).

CATCH STANCE. The full snatch is usually caught in a deep squat, just as with the full clean. The catching stance is the same for both lifts: feet about shoulder-width apart. Just as with the clean, if you can't get below parallel in your squat or aren't able to keep the PVC pipe over the base of your neck at the bottom of your squat, stick to the power snatch and work on your shoulder, upper back, and hip mobility.

HANG POSITION. This is the start position for the snatch's hang variations. It's a little deeper than the clean's hang position because of the wider hand spacing.

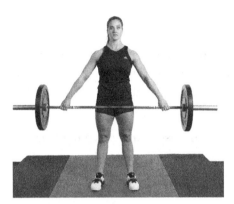

1. With a wide hook grip and elbows straight, hold the bar in the crease of your hip. You should be able to raise your knee without the bar moving.

2. Unlock your knees and push your hips back until the bar is just above your knees.

There's a progression to learning and most people will only need to work on the hang power snatch, starting from above the knees and not worrying about the full snatch for the same reason most people don't need to do a full clean.

The progression follows the same steps as the clean with the addition of the overhead squat:

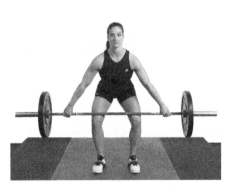

Overhead Squat (page 119)

Snatch High Pull (page 122)

Muscle Snatch (page 123)

Hang Power Snatch (page 130)

Power Snatch from the Floor (page 133)

Hang Snatch & Squat (page 135)

Hang Snatch (page 136)

Full Snatch (page 138)

Overhead Squat

The overhead squat is a great way to improve mobility and stability in the shoulder, mid-back, and hip. Don't begin training the full snatch until your overhead squats are proficient. If your shoulder mobility is really bad or asymmetrical, stick to cleans until you get your shoulders and upper back working properly or you may develop shoulder pain and possible rotator cuff injuries.

You should be able to get your thighs parallel to the floor or lower. Your torso should be vertical, and your arms should be locked out and over the base of your neck. If you can't get there, keep practicing with PVC and do the shoulder mobility exercises daily. Holding the bottom helps open your hips and gets you used to being deep in the squat.

1. Start from the snatch hang position with an unweighted bar.

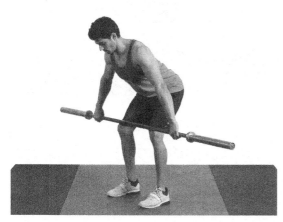

2. Bring the bar overhead with your wrists bent backward and palms facing up; the bar should be resting across your palms, not on your fingertips. Your thumb should now be wrapped around the bar, not in hook grip.

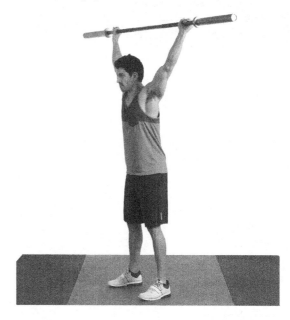

3. Move your feet out so that they're slightly wider than shoulder-width apart and angled out slightly. Sit your hips down and back and go as low as possible while keeping your arms vertical and torso upright. Your feet should be flat on the floor with your knees out.

4. Pause for 2 seconds and stand while keeping the bar directly overhead.

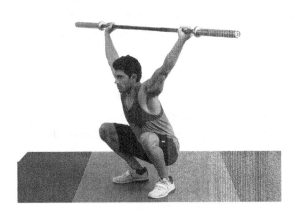

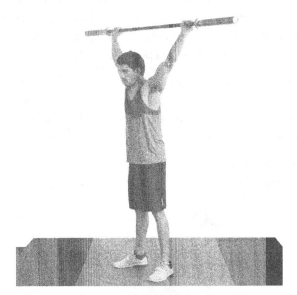

Snatch Pull

This teaches the explosive hip drive and aggressive upward movement of the bar. Remember: This is a practice drill; normally you won't come up on your toes until you're ready to pull yourself under the bar. Don't overemphasize your traps and being on your toes—these parts happen automatically when doing the snatch. Also, the bar path during this stage of training should be almost vertical, though it will move forward slightly as your hips finish their extension.

1. Start from the hang position with an unweighted bar, making sure your elbows are straight at the start of the pull.

2. Drive your hips forward explosively. At the same time, your elbows and head move toward the ceiling and your knees straighten as the bar rides up your thighs. Your elbows float up slightly and your shoulders rise using your traps; you should be coming up onto the toes, but don't hang there.

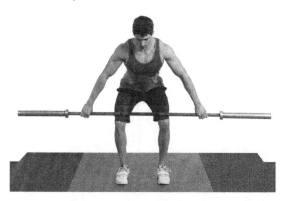

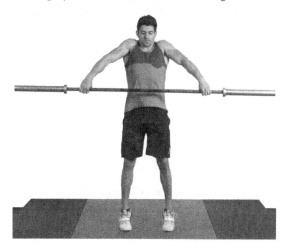

3. As soon as the hip extension is complete, drop back to hang position.

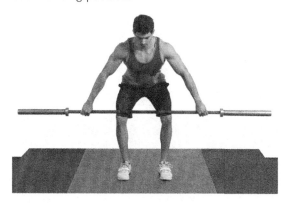

Snatch High Pull

This is the same as the clean High Pull (page 89) but with wider hand spacing.

1. Start from the hang position with an unweighted bar, elbows straight.

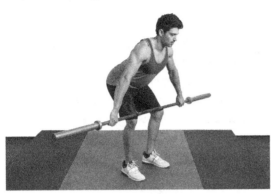

2. Drive your hips forward explosively. Your knees straighten and your torso comes up. As the bar rises from momentum, bend your elbows out to the sides, allowing the bar to rise to about chest level. This is the scarecrow (high pull) position.

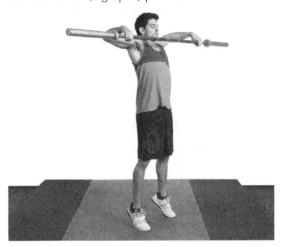

3. To return to hang position, let the bar drop down, pushing your hips back and allowing your knees to bend a little to absorb the energy of the bar.

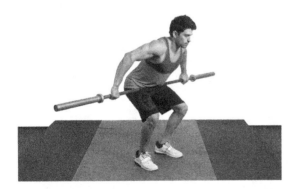

Muscle Snatch

1. Start in hang position using a snatch-width hook grip.

2. Using your arms, pull the bar up, keeping it close to your body.

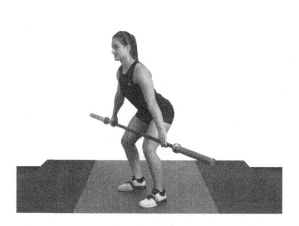

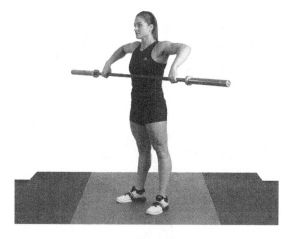

3. Once your elbows have been lifted as high as possible, start to straighten them to bring the bar overhead.

4. Lock your elbows.

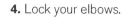

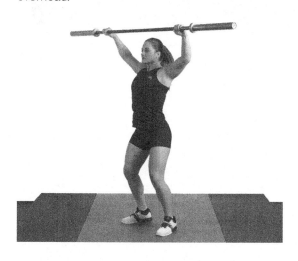

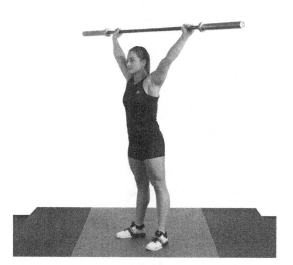

Snatch from the Scarecrow

The snatch from the scarecrow position teaches you how to coordinate the bar going up while you drop under the bar. It's the same position as we worked from in the clean; the only difference is the wider hand spacing on the hook grip.

1. Hold an unweighted bar at chest level with your elbows up (the top position of the snatch high pull) and feet in pulling stance.

2. Punch your hands up to the sky and simultaneously drop under the bar into a partial squat. The bar should be directly over the base of your neck, while your feet remain in the pulling stance.

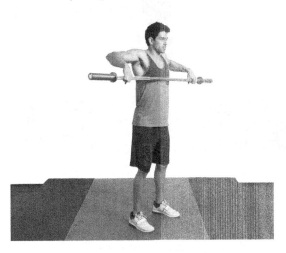

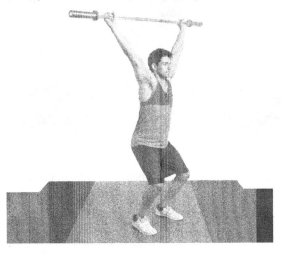

3. Stand up. Once your hips and knees are locked out, bring the bar down to chest level.

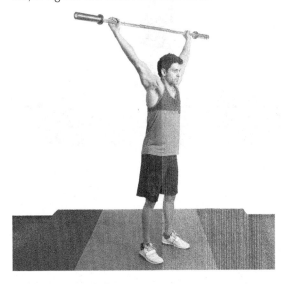

4. Quickly drive your feet out to the catch stance and punch your hands to the ceiling, keeping the bar close to your head. As your feet reconnect with the floor, your elbows should be locked and knees slightly bent.

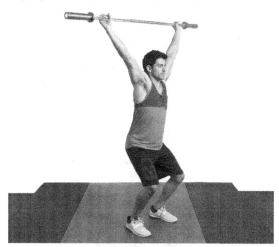

5. Perform an Overhead Squat (page 119).

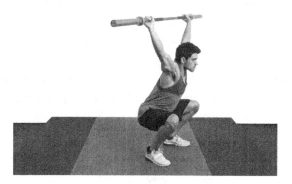

Snatch First Pull

The wide grip requires a deeper stance and stimulates the muscles differently than a deadlift using a standard hand width, making the feel of this move foreign to most lifters. The wider grip forces you to open your hips and engage your lats and upper back more in order to keep your shoulders in their sockets and your back at the proper angle. Just as with the clean, you should work on pulling to various heights with a distinct pause. This helps strengthen any weaknesses in your hips, legs, and back.

1. Position your feet under the bar so that the bar is slightly forward of the knots in your shoelaces.

2. Place your hands on your thighs and push your hips back, allowing your hands to slide to your knees with your elbows straight. This is called the short-stop position.

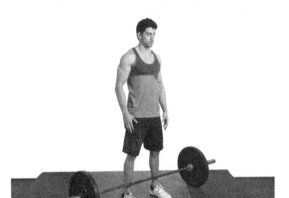

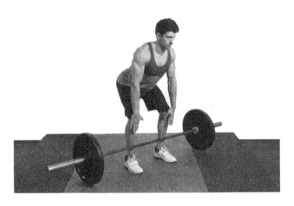

3. From the short-stop position, squat down to the bar and hold with a snatch grip. Your torso should be about 30–35 degrees above horizontal.

4. Drive your knees back and lift your hips and torso together; your torso should remain at 30–35 degrees above horizontal.

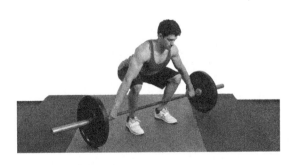

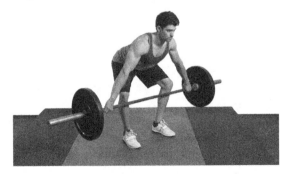

5. Once the bar passes your knees, quickly drive your hips forward and stand up, locking out your hips and knees. You should be standing tall with the bar at your hip crease.

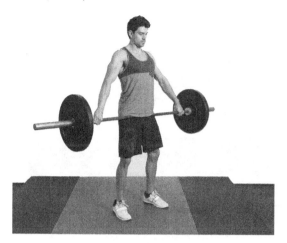

6. Slightly relax your knees and push your hips back.

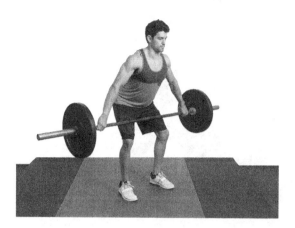

7. As the bar goes below your knees, drop your hips down and squat the bar back to the floor with control.

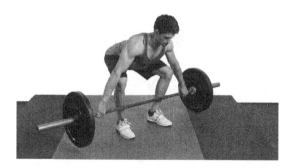

Halting Deadlift

1. Set up as you did in the Snatch-Grip Conventional Deadlift (page 142).

2. Do the snatch grip deadlift and pause 1–2 seconds with the bar 2 inches off the floor.

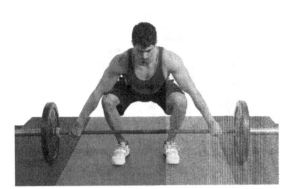

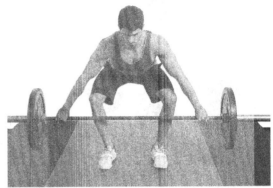

3. Lower the bar to the floor. Do another snatch grip deadlift and pause 1 second with the bar 2 inches off the floor then pull the bar up to your knees and pause for 1 second.

4. Lower the bar to the floor. Do another snatch grip deadlift and pause 1 second with the bar 2 inches off the floor then pull the bar up to your knee and pause for 1 second. Continue to pull the bar until it's above your knee and pause again for 1 second.

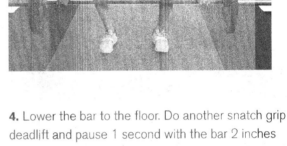

5. Lower the bar, pausing at the same spots for the same duration as you did on the way up. Do another snatch grip deadlift and pause 1 second with the bar 2 inches off the floor, then pull the bar up to your knees and pause for 1 second. Continue to pull the bar until it's above your knee and pause again for 1 second. Finally, pull the bar up to mid-thigh and pause for 1 second.

6. Lower the bar, pausing at the same spots for the same duration as you did on the way up.

7. Finally, repeat steps 1–6 but finish with your knees and hips locked out with the bar across your hip crease. Then lower it the same as before.

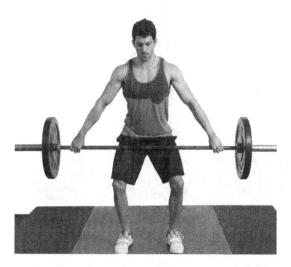

Hang Power Snatch

The only difference between this and the hang snatch and squat is that you should squat while catching the bar instead of catching then squatting.

1. Start from the hang position with an unweighted bar.

2. Drive your hips forward explosively and straighten your knees, keeping the bar against your thighs.

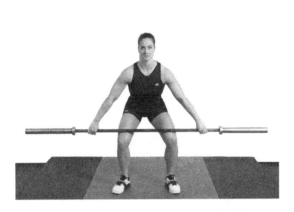

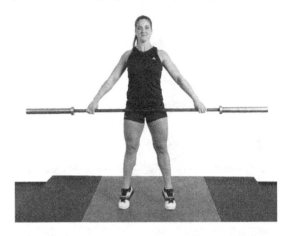

3. You should find yourself rising up and the bar coming up to chest level, elbows up.

4. Quickly drive your feet out to the catch stance and punch your hands to the ceiling. Your elbows should lock out as your feet reconnect with the floor. As your feet land, your knees should bend so that you're absorbing the force of the bar with your legs.

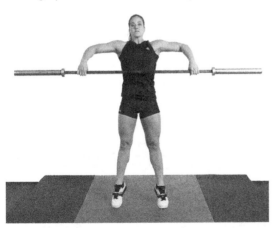

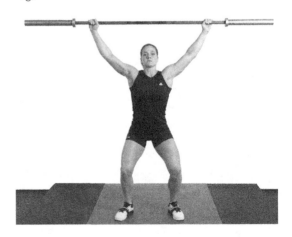

As with the jerk, you're trying to get under the bar once it's at chest level. Get under the bar; do *not* press the bar overhead. Remember, the bar should not travel forward away from your body or head.

When the hang snatch feels good, start with the bar higher up on your thighs, which forces you to develop more explosive power in your hips. Other variations to develop more power include starting from jerk blocks positioned just above the knees in the hang position. Because the bar is resting on the boxes, you won't be able to pre-load the body; basically, you're starting dead in the water. This means you'll have to go lighter, but it will make the lift much more powerful and faster.

Two-Phase Snatch

This breaks the full power snatch into two pieces to teach the first pull and to work the transition from the first pull to the second pull.

1. Perform the first pull, stopping in the hang position at mid-thigh. Pause 2 to 3 seconds.

2. Perform a Hang Power Snatch (page 130).

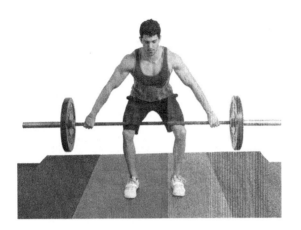

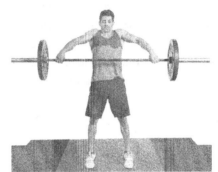

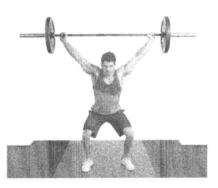

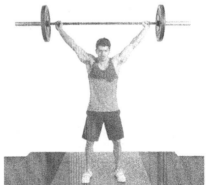

Doing the halting deadlift and the two-phase snatch reinforces proper body positioning through the various phases of the snatch. Over time, reduce the pause in the two-phase snatch until it's eliminated, at which point you'll do either the power snatch from the floor or the full snatch.

Power Snatch from the Floor

The starting position for this move is deeper than the power clean because of the wider hand spacing on the bar. Therefore, you must have a lot better hip mobility to get into position.

Start with PVC or a junior Olympic bar and light training plates. If you use PVC, you'll need to be able to rest it on low blocks so that it's the same distance from the floor as a loaded bar.

1. Start in the short-stop position.

2. Squat down to the bar and position your hands into a wide hook grip. Your torso should be about 30–35 degrees above horizontal.

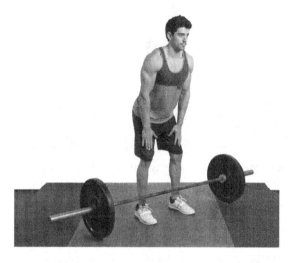

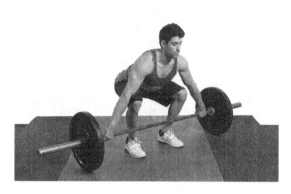

3. Drive your knees back and lift your hips and torso together; your torso should still be at 30–35 degrees above horizontal.

4. Once the bar passes your knees, quickly drive your hips forward and pull the bar to chest level.

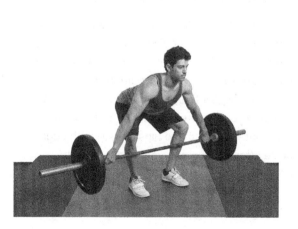

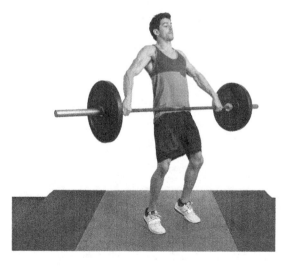

5. As your elbows rise and the bar comes to chest level, quickly drive your feet out to the catch stance and get under the bar quickly, dropping into a partial squat while punching your hands toward the sky. Your elbows should be locked out as your feet plant.

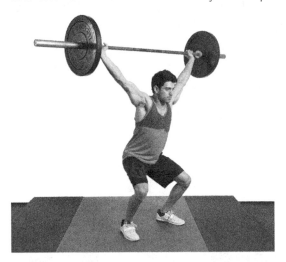

6. Stand up.

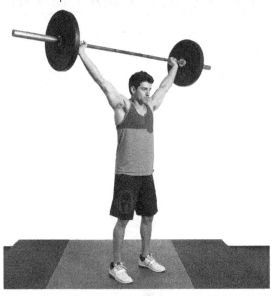

There are actually two ways to finish the set-up and start the first pull. In the first, known as a static start, you do as described above: Push your hips back until your hands are knee level and then squat to the bar, grab it, lift your chest, and pull. This is good for beginners and those trying to develop more power by eliminating the stretch-shortening cycle. The stretch shortening, which happens in the second variation called the dynamic start, creates more power by releasing and regaining tension. It's similar to bouncing out of the bottom of a squat.

With the dynamic start, everything is the same as the static start, but once you have your hands on the bar, you'll lift your hips up, keeping your torso in the same place, then drop your hips back down and immediately go into the first pull. This "pumping" action of your hips reloads them. You must make sure that your torso and hips are still in the right place after the pump or your first pull will be negatively impacted.

Hang Snatch & Squat

Doing the snatch and squat allows you to work each part individually if you're having problems getting under the bar. It also helps train the overhead squat as a separate movement, though you'll integrate the two soon. Pay close attention to the path of the bar as it moves through "scarecrow" position (high pull) to overhead. The bar's path should be almost vertical. Since you're pulling vertically when you drop under the bar, it should move out slightly. Just make sure you aren't flipping your forearms out in front.

1. Start from the hang position with an unweighted bar.

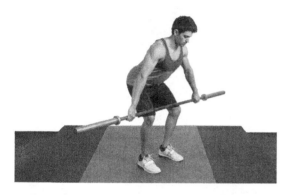

2. Drive your hips forward and straighten your knees, keeping the bar against your thighs. You should find yourself rising up and the bar coming up to chest level, elbows up. Your elbows and body rise as the bar moves to chest level.

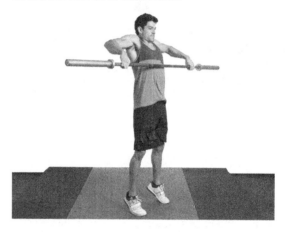

3. Quickly drive your feet out to the catch stance and punch your hands to the ceiling, keeping the bar close to your head. As your feet reconnect with the floor, your elbows should be locked and knees slightly bent.

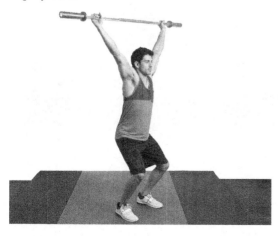

4. Perform an Overhead Squat (page 119).

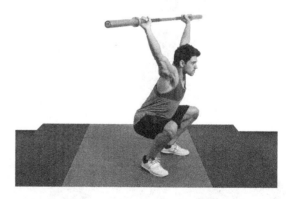

Hang Snatch

Keep in mind that this is a very fast, fluid movement.

1. Hold the barbell using a snatch-width hook grip in the hang position.

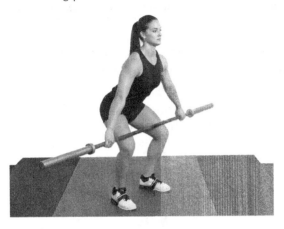

2. Explosively drive your hips forward and pull the bar to chest level, keeping the bar close to your body.

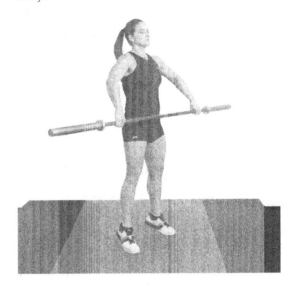

3. As the bar reaches chest level, finish extending your hips and knees. At this point you should be on your toes.

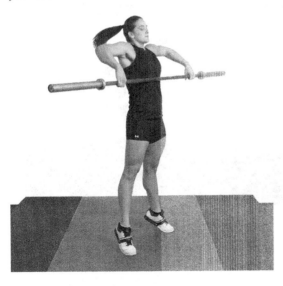

4. Quickly drive your feet out to catch stance, pull yourself under the bar and drop into a full squat while allowing your arms to straighten overhead.

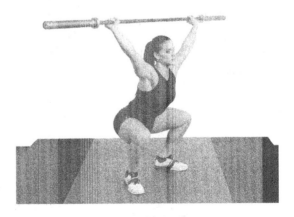

5. Stand tall, keeping the bar overhead.

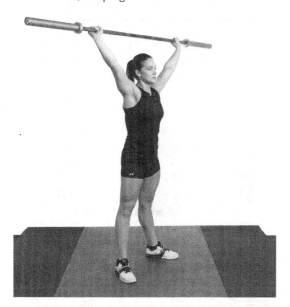

Full Snatch

1. Set up and initiate the first pull as you did in the Power Snatch from the Floor (page 133).

2. As the bar reaches mid-thigh, drive your hips and knees forward, bring your head up, and get the bar to chest level (scarecrow position).

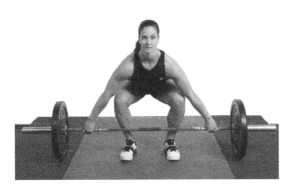

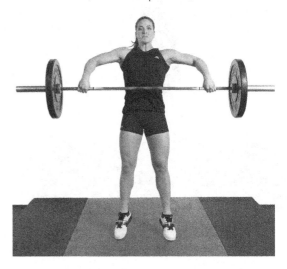

3. Quickly drive your feet out to your catch stance, pulling yourself under the bar while punching your hands toward the ceiling and straightening your elbows. As your feet plant on the floor, drop into a deep squat while simultaneously catching the bar overhead with your elbows locked out. This is a continuous movement.

4. Stand up, keeping the bar over the base of your neck.

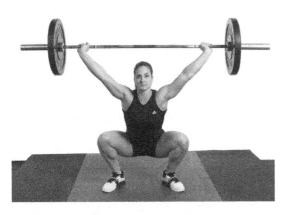

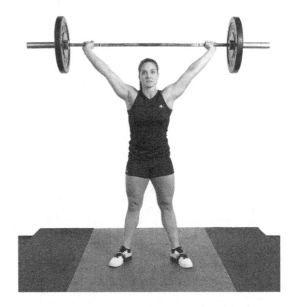

Standing is one place where lifters lose the lift. A slight forward or backward deviation coming out of the squat will cause you to lose control of a heavier bar. If you do lose the bar, let it fall in the direction it wants to and quickly move the other way. For example, if you lose it to the front, push it forward, away from you, and step back. If you lose it behind you, let it fall and quickly move forward. This is why your lifting area must be free of obstructions.

If the weight on the bar is light, bring it back to your chest and control its descent to the floor. If it's heavy or you're fatigued, let the bar fall from overhead but maintain hand contact with the bar to control where it goes. The bar will bounce (you're using bumper plates, right?) so be ready to move or use your hands to deflect it.

Some people will also do the split snatch, which is performing a hang snatch or snatch from the floor and catching it in the split position (the same stance as the split jerk). See page 150 to see how to get into a split stance properly.

Full Snatch with Split Stance

The split stance is a nice change of pace. It works the hips in a different plane and range of motion. It also gives more stability front to back so that you're less likely to lose the bar behind you when standing. However, you may not be able to lift as much weight because you won't be able to get under the bar as deeply.

1. Set up based on whether you'll be doing the split snatch from the hang or from the floor.

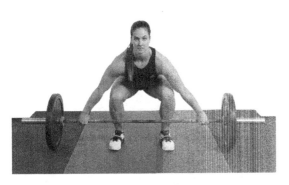

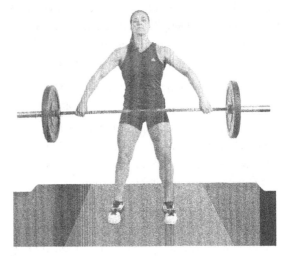

2. Initiate the snatch.

3. As the bar gets to chest level, drive one leg forward and one back and get under the bar as fast as possible. The front shin should be vertical, while the back leg will be somewhat bent. Your arms should lock out as you settle into the split.

4. Stand up and bring your rear foot forward, your front foot backward, or a little of both.

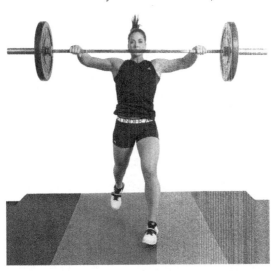

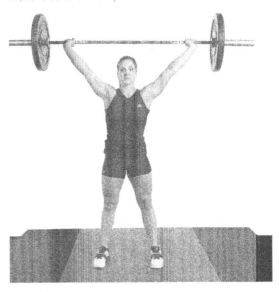

PART 4
ASSISTANCE LIFTS

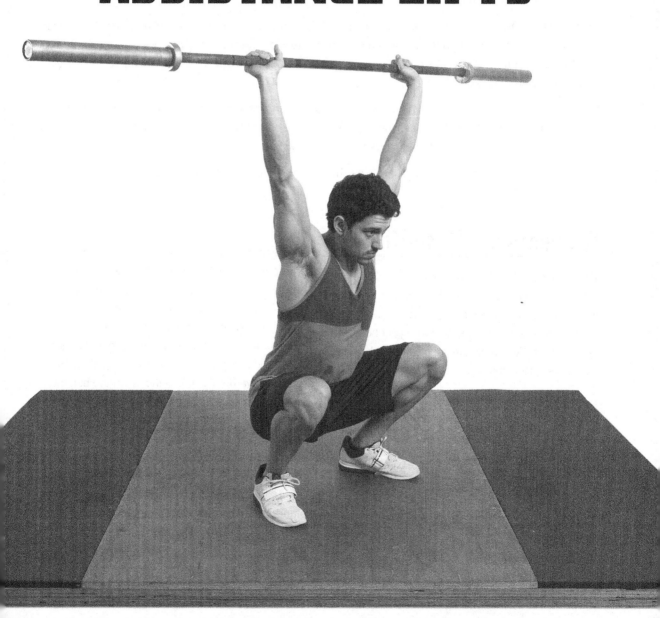

Assistance lifts help train specific areas associated with the primary Olympic lift movements. For example, front, back, and goblet squats are assistance lifts for the full clean and full snatch. Overhead shrugs are an assistance exercise for the overhead position in both the snatch and the jerk.

DEADLIFT

The first pull in both the snatch and the clean aren't exactly deadlifts but deadlifts are similar enough that we want to target them in order to help build strength. (In addition, practice the first pull movement that's described on page 98 and page 126.) Use standard Olympic plates or training plates so that the bar will be the correct distance from the floor. There are several deadlift variations but we'll focus on the two most common: the conventional deadlift and the Romanian deadlift (RDL).

BODY POSITION. As you train using these variations, you'll also want to work with different grip widths. Since the hand placement on the bar in the snatch is very wide, you'll want to practice deadlifts with a wide grip to get used to it and build strength in your back with your arms out wide. The hand position for cleans and deadlifts are the same.

Hand placement on the bar should be such that your arms hang straight down from your shoulder blades and your hands are just outside the shins. The grip can be done one of two ways: with your hands wrapped over the bar (double overhand) or with a hook grip (see page 83).

Your chin should be tucked as though you were holding a ping-pong ball with it. Maintain that head position for both deadlift variations.

Conventional Deadlift

This variation targets your glutes and secondarily your quads and hamstrings. Your entire torso must remain locked with a neutral spine all the way up and back down. Do *not* look forward with your head—this causes excessive arching in your lower back and can cause disc problems.

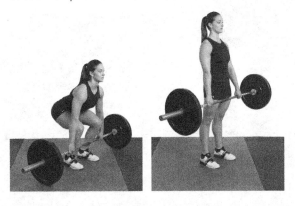

1. Approach the bar with your feet hip-width or slightly wider apart. The bar should be over your mid-foot, about where your shoelaces are tied; it will be an inch or so from your shins. Push your hips back, let your knees bend slightly, reach straight down, and place your hands on the bar using the overhand or hook grip. Your hands should be just outside your legs. Once you set your grip, push your knees forward until your shins touch the bar, then lift your chest up. Your lower back should be flat or slightly arched. Your shoulders will be in front of the bar but there should be a straight line from your scapulae to the bar. Looking at it from the side, a line drawn from your shoulder blade through your arm to the bar should be perfectly vertical. **2.** To stand up, straighten your knees and move your hips forward. As the bar moves up past your knees, your torso comes up. Keep your arms straight throughout the lift; don't try to lift the bar with your arms by bending your elbows. As you stand, keep the bar in close—you should be literally pulling the bar up your shins and maintaining contact as it comes up your thighs. Also make sure not to straighten your knees before the bar is above them. If your knees straighten out too soon, your hips will come up too quickly, which can cause back issues. At the top position standing fully upright, your glutes, hamstrings, quads, core, and grip should be locked out. Everything should be tight even if the weight is light for you.

Reverse the movement to put the bar on the floor. Stay tight as you lower the bar; don't let your lower back round.

Romanian Deadlift (RDL)

The Romanian deadlift hits the hamstrings more than anything else, but the movement is essentially the same as the conventional version. The primary difference is the knee bend. In the RDL your knees are "soft"—your knees barely bend as your hips go straight back but not down.

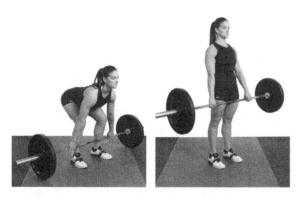

1. Approach the bar with your feet hip-width or slightly wider apart. The bar should be over your mid-foot, about where your shoelaces are tied; it will be an inch or so from your shins. **2.** Push your hips back, let your knees bend slightly, reach straight

down, and place your hands on the bar using the overhand or hook grip. Your hands should be just outside your legs. Once you set your grip, lift your chest up. Your lower back should be flat or slightly arched. Your shoulders will be in front of the bar but there should be a straight line from your scapulae to the bar. Looking at it from the side, a line drawn from your shoulder blade through your arm to the bar should be perfectly vertical. **3.** To stand up, keep your knees relaxed and move your hips forward. As the bar moves up past your knees, your torso comes up. Keep your arms straight throughout the lift; don't try to lift the bar with your arms by bending your elbows. As you stand, keep the bar in close—you should be literally pulling the bar up your shins and maintaining contact as it comes up your thighs. Also make sure not to fully straighten your knees before the bar is above them. If your knees straighten out too soon, your hips will come up too quickly, which can cause back issues. **4.** At the top position standing fully upright, your glutes, hamstrings, quads, knees, core, and grip should be locked out. Everything should be tight even if the weight is light for you.

To lower the bar, push your hips back and let the bar lightly touch your thighs as it goes down. Let your knees bend as the bar goes below them, allowing you to bend and push your hips back farther. Keep pushing your hips back without bending your knees anymore until the bar is on the floor.

SNATCH GRIP VARIATION: Set up just as you did with the conventional deadlift, except use a snatch-width grip. Make sure you practice the Snatch First Pull (page 126) and the Clean First Pull (page 98) as described in their respective sections.

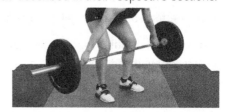

SQUATS

In Olympic weightlifting, we don't really differentiate between types of squats. A squat is a movement pattern, not an exercise—the only difference is where the load is placed: rack position, backs of the shoulders, or, when using a kettlebell, a goblet or front squat. There's even a bodyweight squat. Regardless of which you do, the movement pattern should be the same.

Powerlifters' and most other trainees' front squat with the bar in rack looks totally different from the squat with the bar on the backs of the shoulder or lower down on the back. The front squat is always with a vertical torso; to do otherwise means you'll probably drop the bar or fall over face first. With the back squat, the torso is angled forward, which keeps the bar centered over the feet and helps keep you from dropping the bar behind you or falling backward. A lot of that is due to the extreme loads powerlifters are squatting—700 pounds or more! With practice, developing a strong core, and improving your hip flexibility, you should be able to do any squat with an upright torso.

Olympic lifters use a shoe with a raised heel. These are specifically designed for Olympic weightlifting and the heel height can vary but is typically ¾ inch. These shoes are very solid, giving you a strong base of support. The elevation helps keep the torso vertical, especially if you have limited range of motion in your ankles and hips. The shoes can make a huge difference in your squats, so if you plan on doing Olympic weightlifting, I highly recommend you get a pair. A decent shoe runs about $100 per pair. Do-Win's and Sabo are good brands. You'll have to search around online because you probably won't find them at your sporting-goods store. Pay attention to sizing recommendations so that you get the right size the first time.

While most cross-training and running shoes have elevated heels that are designed to cushion your feet and absorb energy, this is exactly the opposite of what we need. Olympic weightlifting shoes transmit all of your force from the floor into the bar and provide you with a solid, stable surface. Running shoes and other cross-trainers won't.

If you don't have Olympic weightlifting shoes yet, you can get the feel of them by placing a ¾-inch board under your heels—just make sure it can't slide around. This is a simulation, not a replacement, of the proper shoes, and should be used only for squats. To use the board, begin by doing a few bodyweight squats barefoot with your feet flat on the floor. Check your position: Your torso should be vertical with no forward lean, your knees aligned with your toes, and thighs at or below parallel. Now place your heels on the ¾-inch board with the mid-portion of your feet off the board and the balls of your feet to your toes on the floor. Perform a few more squats with the board and observe any differences in your torso and shin position in comparison to the bodyweight squat with your feet on the floor. If your torso is vertical and your shins nearly so, your ankles and hips are restricting your squat and you should get a pair of Olympic lifting shoes.

While using the board for squats is fine, do not use it when doing cleans or snatches. There's too much risk. If you cannot perform a proper squat, you shouldn't do the full lifts.

When adding load (weights) to the squat, the barbell can be held in rack position, behind the neck on the shoulders, or overhead. The squat movement remains the same regardless of whether you're doing a bodyweight, front, or goblet squat, but where you hold your load determines the difficulty level and which muscles are used.

Bodyweight Squat

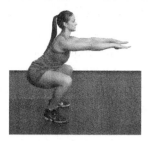

1. Start with your feet about shoulder-width apart and turned outward just a little, no more than 15–20 degrees. Reach your hands out in front of you at shoulder height; this helps with balance. **2.** Activating your hip flexors, push your hips down and back, keeping your shins vertical as your knees bend. Your weight should be on the mid-portion of your feet, back to your heels, and also along the outside edges of your feet—think "heels down, instep up." Keep your spine neutral, chin tucked. Go as low as you can without your tailbone rounding under. **3.** Once at the bottom, stay tight and drive back up through your heels, maintaining the heels-down, instep-up foot position. Don't bounce out of the bottom; it will cause you to lose control and allows your core to deactivate. If you got below parallel, you should feel your glutes as well as your quads working.

Barbell Front Squat

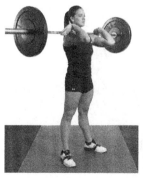
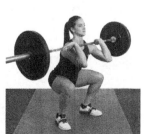

1. Do a Power Clean from the Floor (page 103) to bring the bar to rack position. If using a squat rack, set the hooks at shoulder level and place your bar on the hooks. Get under the bar and into rack position. **2.** Sit down into your hips just as you did with the bodyweight squat, keeping your torso tall and spine neutral. Don't let your tailbone tuck under. Keep your upper arms parallel to the floor. **3.** Once you've reached your depth, drive through your heels and stand.

Barbell Back Squat

Depending on the load, you may clean and jerk the bar overhead then lower it onto the backs of your shoulders or use a squat rack with the hooks set to shoulder height, with the bar on the hooks.

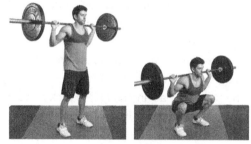

1. Step backward and position the bar across your trapezius. Stick out your chest and try to bend the bar across your back. Keep your traps and lats tight. **2.** Pull your hips back and down and try to keep your upper body as close to vertical as possible. The depth of your squat depends on your flexibility. You should try to get your thighs parallel to your hips or lower while maintaining proper knee and foot tracking; however, don't allow your lower back to round. **3.** Drive through your heels and return to standing. Keep your entire midsection tight, not just your belly. Create a belt around your body by breathing into your entire lower back and sides as well as your abs.

When you're done, walk back to the rack and place the bar back on the hooks.

Sots Press

The Sots Press is a variation that works on stability at the bottom of the squat as well as pressing strength and shoulder/upper-back mobility and stability.

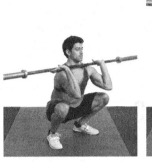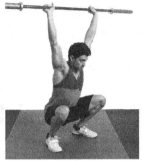

1. Perform a Barbell Front Squat (page 145). At the bottom of the squat, drop your elbows down. **2.** Move your head back a bit and press the bar overhead. Once your elbows are locked out, move your head forward through your arms. Other than your hand placement, this is the same position as the bottom of the snatch. **3.** You can stand up with the bar overhead and bring it to rack position, or bring it to the backs of the shoulders.

Goblet Squat

The Goblet Squat is a great assistance lift. It teaches all the mechanics of the upright torso and proper hip and knee movement without having to deal with being able to maintain a good rack position.

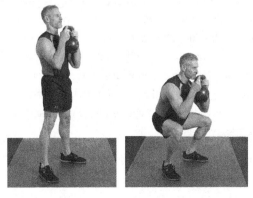

1. Hold a kettlebell with both hands by its "horns" at sternum level. The bell will be close to your body but not touching, and your elbows should be down. **2.** Keeping your torso upright and elbows in and down, squeeze your abs and pull yourself down with your hip flexors. Try to get your hips below your knees if possible, but don't compromise your structure by tipping over, letting your knees collapse, or otherwise losing form. If you have the flexibility in your hips and lower back, try to get your butt to your calves. Squat as deeply as your ability allows. Pause at the bottom and use your elbows to pry your hips open a little. **3.** Drive through your heels and stand up.

DUMBBELL VARIATION: The only difference when using a dumbbell is how it's held. Pick the dumbbell up and hold it vertically, placing the top end in the palms of both hands, which are facing up.

Kettlebell Front Squat

Also called a kettlebell rack squat, this version has you place a kettlebell in rack position and squat. Heavy kettlebell front squats are a great exercise to train the lateral stabilizers. No side bending or rotation is allowed during the movement so you have to engage your obliques and other stabilizers.

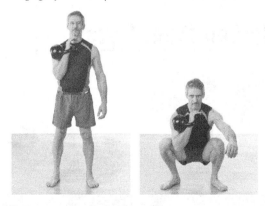

1. Start with the bell in rack position (elbow is in tight against your ribs, wrist is straight but relaxed, forearm is leaning slightly inward toward your body) and your feet in squat stance. **2.** Keeping your torso upright, squeeze your abs and pull yourself down with your hip flexors. Try to get your hips below your knees if possible, but don't compromise your structure by tipping over, letting your knees collapse, or otherwise losing form. If you have the flexibility in your hips and lower back, try to get your butt to your calves. Squat as deeply as your ability allows. **3.** Drive through your heels and stand up.

Perform reps on both sides.

If you find the bell is falling off your forearm, you're either rotating your torso during the squat, leaning forward, or not holding it correctly.

DOUBLE KETTLEBELL VARIATION: You can also do the front squat with two bells, one in each hand. However, the second bell balances you out so you no longer have to stabilize being pulled to the side, meaning your obliques aren't working as hard. You can train this exercise with a heavy bell on one side and a lighter one on the other, which feels different at first but makes you work harder. It's a great way to teach your body how to deal with uneven loads. *Note:* Do not attempt this variation unless you can do a Kettlebell Double Dead Clean (see below), the only safe way to get two bells into rack.

Kettlebell Double Dead Clean

A rather technical lift that develops a lot of power, this is a great exercise in and of itself. The movement looks very similar to a barbell clean, but there are some significant differences—most notably the rack

positions are totally different. If you rack a kettlebell the same way as a bar, you'll destroy your wrists.

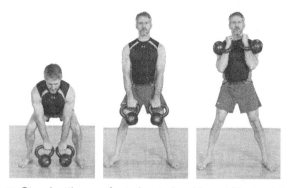

1. Stand with your feet about shoulder-width apart and the bell on the floor between your feet, angling the handle back. With each arm hanging straight and your torso upright, squat down and grab the handles of both bells so that the webbing between your thumb and forefinger faces your feet. Look out, not down. Sink your hips and keep your torso upright. **2–3.** Driving through your heels, explode straight up. Your shoulders should naturally rise from the hip explosion as the bells come up. Using the upward momentum, let your arms and the bells continue to rise. As the bells reach approximately chest height, drop your elbows and drive your hands up through the handles. Keep your elbows in close. **4.** Once you've cleaned the bells, squat just as you've been doing. **5–6.** To put the bells down, bump your elbows a little and bend your wrists so that your fingers point to the floor; let the bells fall off your forearms into your fingers. As this happens, straighten your arms and sink your hips down, allowing your legs to absorb the force of the bells. The bells should lightly touch the floor. The end position is the same as the start.

KETTLEBELL SNATCHES

Like kettlebell cleans, kettlebell snatches differ from the barbell version when lifting the weight overhead. While I've focused on just the dead snatch here, there are many variations; see my other Ulysses Press book *The Ultimate Kettlebell Workbook* for details on the other types of kettlebell snatches.

Both these snatch variations along with the dead cleans (page 147) help develop the explosive hip power that's needed in the barbell snatch. The snatch can also be used as conditioning (i.e., doing higher reps), which isn't recommended with the bar version.

One-Arm Kettlebell Dead Snatch

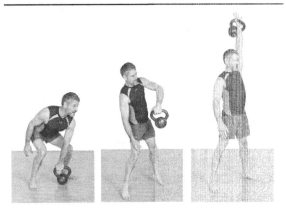

1. Stand with your feet between hip- and shoulder-width apart. Place the kettlebell on the floor between your feet. Using your right hand, rotate the handle so that it's at a 45-degree angle to your body; the front corner of the bell will be angled to the right. Grab the REAR corner of the bell by wrapping your right thumb and fingers around the handle.   **2–3.** Keeping your arm as close to your body as possible without the bell hitting you, explode straight up and pull the bell off the floor. The bell's path is vertical. Keep your thumb pointed toward you as the bell comes up. As your hips extend, your shoulder rises, followed by your elbow, forearm, wrist, hand, and bell. When your hips are fully extended, your right shoulder should be at its highest point and your elbow should be higher than your shoulder.   **4.** As your forearm continues upward, your elbow straightens. When your forearm approaches vertical, flip your wrist so that your fingers point up. The bell should rotate around your wrist. Hold the overhead position briefly, making sure that your elbow and knees are locked out.   **5.** To return the bell to the floor, quickly bend your wrist so that your fingers point to the floor. As the bell comes off your hand, bend your elbow and let the bell fall into the crook of your fingers. Wrap your thumb over your index finger and rotate your forearm so that your thumb points to your centerline; your thumb and forefinger take the brunt of the weight.   **6–7.** As the bell falls, straighten out your right arm and squat down, matching the speed of the bell with your legs so that your arm is straight when the bell lightly touches the floor. Keep your torso vertical. Use your legs to slow the bell, not your arm. The descent should be as smooth and fluid as the ascent of the bell. *Note:* There should be no jerking of the arm; it should not be used as a brake. The legs are doing all the work.

You won't catch the kettlebell snatch with bent knees unless it's very heavy. In those cases, a slight knee bend to get under the bell is acceptable. If you use the knee bend, stand up after the elbow locks out.

DOUBLE KETTLEBELL VARIATION: Do not do the double bell version until you've repeatedly practiced the one-arm dead snatch to proficiency. The double is the same as the one-arm version except you're snatching two bells at once, one in each hand.

BOX JUMPS

Box jumps train the lower body for explosive power. While they're a great exercise, don't do high reps, which can lead to torn Achilles tendons. After you've jumped on the box, step down instead of jumping back down. Reversing the jump can also lead to ruptured Achilles tendons.

Always check the integrity of the box before jumping on it. Don't use plates or aerobic steps for jumps—they may shift when you land, causing you to fall. Make sure the box can't slide. Your box should be about the height of your shins, lower if you're new to box jumps and slightly higher if you've done them before. Be smart—I've seen people jumping 5 feet up to very unstable surfaces; that's just asking for trouble. Typically 16-, 18-, 20-, or 24-inch boxes will suffice.

Box Jump

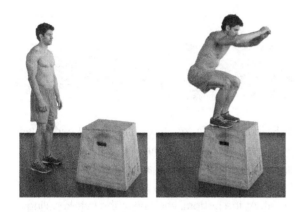

1. Stand about 6–10 inches from a box with your feet comfortably apart, hip to shoulder width. **2.** Quickly push your hips back and down into a quarter squat. Your torso should be angled and your arms should reach back at the same angle as your back. **3–4.** Explode forward—not straight up—so that you land on the box. Use your arms to generate momentum by raising them up in front of you as you jump. At the same time, bring your knees up just enough so that your feet clear the box. Land with the balls of your feet touching the box first, then your heels. Your entire foot, not just the balls of your feet, should be on the box. Try to land softly, like a cat, making little to no noise. Once you've landed, stand up, bringing your hips through. Don't stop short.

Step off the box and return to start position.

LUNGES

Lunges are trained for both overall hip strength and core stability, as well as to improve strength and balance in the split jerk. Jumping lunges also help train foot speed and coordination required for the split jerk. While not exactly the same as the split jerk position, the ability to perform lunges well will greatly enhance your split jerk stance.

Split Squat

This is also called the static lunge.

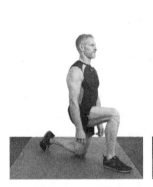 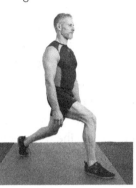

1. Get into the half-kneeling position. Your front thigh should be parallel to the floor and your front shin should be vertical. **2.** With an upright torso and your hips under you, squeeze your abs, glutes, and quads, drive off your front heel, and stand tall. Your front knee won't lock out but your back knee will. Keep your torso vertical at all times, with your hips under your shoulders and your spine neutral. Don't lean forward.

Return to start position. Switch sides.

Forward Lunge

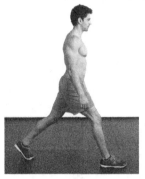 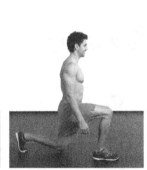

1. Stand with your feet hip-width apart. Leading with your heel, step forward with one leg; the distance should be a little longer than your normal stride length. **2.** Sink your hips straight down into a lunge. At the bottom, you'll be in the half-kneeling position. Your feet should be in line with their respective hips and your hips should be under your shoulders with no forward or backward lean. Your lead shin is always vertical. Don't lean forward when doing this move. **3.** Driving through your front heel, come up tall, and step your lead foot back to start position.

Switch sides. Step back then repeat with the other foot.

Reverse Lunge

The reverse lunge can be tricky—proper foot placement is important. If you step too far backward, you'll be unable to keep your hips under your shoulders. If you don't step back far enough, you won't have room to sink down. Many people lean forward as they reach the foot backward, which works your quads hard but can aggravate your knees. To work your glutes more and make your core stronger, try to keep your torso upright and move from your hips.

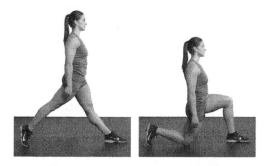

1. Stand with your feet hip-width apart. Step backward with one foot until you're in the exact same position as the top of the Split Squat (page 150). **2.** Staying tight, sink your hips down. Try to keep your torso upright at all times—think about someone pulling you from a rope or band wrapped around your hips. **3.** Drive through your front heel to come up and step forward, bringing your feet back together.

Switch sides.

Jumping Lunge

This jumping version has you quickly switching your legs at the top of the movement. Land softly like a cat.

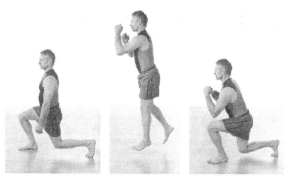

1. Assume a 90/90 position. **2.** Come up quickly, keeping your torso vertical. As you come up, lift your back foot off the floor briefly then re-bend your lead knee. Your back foot shouldn't be pushing off—all the work is being done by your lead leg, focusing on your hip. As you reach the top position, quickly bring your back leg forward and your lead leg back. Be soft on your landing like a cat.

OVERHEAD PRESSES

We've talked about pressing while practicing snatches with an unweighted bar and PVC but you should also use the overhead barbell press to build strength in your shoulders, back, and core.

Barbell Overhead Press

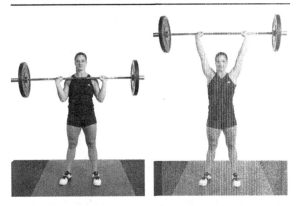

1. Clean the bar to rack position, then lower your elbows and close your hands around the bar with your wrists bent back, palms facing up.   **2.** With your feet under your hips or slightly wider, exhale and contract your body to drive the bar up, keeping everything tight. Pull your head back slightly as the bar goes straight up.   **3.** As your arms extend overhead, stick your head forward through your arms. Don't bend your knees. Lock your elbows and inhale at the top.   **4.** With control, exhale and lower the bar back to your collar bones, moving your head back a little as the bar comes down.

Barbell Behind-the-Neck Press

If you have shoulder or neck problems, you should avoid this lift. You can either clean the bar and perform a standard press and bring the bar behind your neck or place the bar in a squat rack (like during the Barbell Back Squat, page 145).

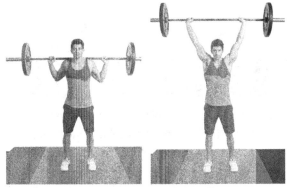

1. Once the bar is across the back of your traps, brace as we described in the Barbell Overhead Press.   **2.** Push your head forward slightly to get it out of the way and exhale as you press the bar. Don't bend your knees. Lock your elbows and inhale at the top.   **3.** With control, exhale and lower the bar back behind the backs of your shoulders. Don't allow the bar to drop.

If you lose control, let the bar fall whichever way it wants while you quickly move the other way.

OTHER FUNDAMENTAL EXERCISES

Whether you practice Olympic weightlifting or not, these are fundamental movements will help you move better and get stronger overall.

Push-Up

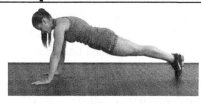

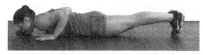

1. Start with your hands shoulder-width apart and your arms straight. Spread your fingers so that the middle fingers point straight ahead and the first and third finger on the right hand point to 11 and 1 o'clock and the reverse on the left; this helps spread the stress across the entire hand rather than put it in the wrist. Push the floor away so that your shoulder blades aren't sticking out. You should be on the balls of your feet with your feet no more than shoulder-width apart. Keep your quads, glutes, and abs locked tight. There should be a straight line from the base of your neck to your heels—don't lift your butt up or let it sag.   **2.** Slowly lower yourself down, pointing your elbows to the rear, not to the sides. At the bottom position, your triceps and lats should touch.

Return to the top position, making sure you're actively pushing the floor away.

MODIFICATION: If you can't maintain a plank position, elevate your hands on a stable surface that's high enough to allow you to do a proper push-up. Over time, decrease the height of the platform and keep practicing; eventually you'll be able to do them on the floor.

Spiderman Push-Up

These require a lot more core and shoulder strength/ stability than standard push-ups.

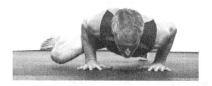

1. From a high plank, lower down for your push-up. As your body gets closer to the floor, pull one knee up toward your elbow on the outside of your body. Your inner thigh should be parallel to the floor.
2. As you drive away from the floor, return the leg to the start position.

On the next rep pull the other knee up.

Quad Press

This is a very springy movement that's a cross between a push-up and a crawl position.

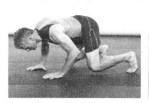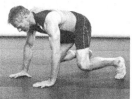

1. Start on hands and knees, with your hands a little wider than your shoulders, your knees slightly behind your hips, and your feet as wide as your hands. Lift your knees off the floor and straighten your elbows. Maintaining neutral spine, keep your back parallel to the floor.   **2.** Bend your elbows and knees and move toward the floor. **3.** Keeping your back parallel to the floor, push away from the floor equally with both hands and feet. When your elbows straighten out, quickly reverse the movement.

Quad Hop

This very dynamic move requires a lot of explosive power from your arms and legs while requiring your core to work extra hard to keep your hips and shoulders level.

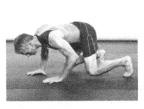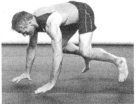

1. Set up like the Quad Press (page 153). **2.** Instead of pushing away from the floor with your hands and feet, explode up. **3.** Land softly, absorbing your body weight into your chest, shoulders, feet, quads, and glutes. Don't land with stiff arms or you'll injure your wrists and shoulders. Your back needs to remain parallel to the floor.

Bootstrapper

The bootstrapper opens the hips, helps loosen up the lower back, and works on ankle mobility.

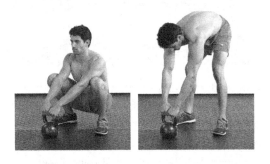

1. Stand with your feet slightly wider than your shoulders and place a bell about 6 inches in front of

them. Inhale then exhale as you grab the bell with both hands and squat deeply, keeping an upright torso and your knees lined up with your toes. Hold onto the bell like an anchor and sit back and down on your heels. Use your elbows to pry your knees apart. Find space in your hips. Hold the exhale for 2 seconds. **2.** Still holding the bell, inhale as you lift your hips up and let your head release to the floor. You're now stretching your hamstrings. Hold for a second and then pull yourself back down.

Do 5 reps.

POST VARIATION: If you don't have a kettlebell, you can use a post instead.

1. Grab a post at waist level. Squat down, keeping your torso and shins vertical. Move backward from the post if necessary to get your shins vertical. Your feet are always flat on the floor. **2.** Go as low as you can without letting your torso fall forward or your knee drive forward past your toes.

Shift a little from side to side then stand back up to start position.

Pull-Up

Pull-ups work the lats and back more than chin-ups.

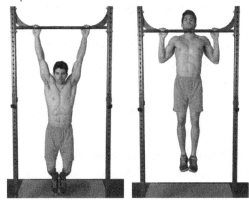

1. Hang from the bar with your hands in line with your shoulders or slightly wider and your palms facing forward. Pack your shoulders in their sockets and allow your legs and elbows to be slightly bent (this keeps tension through the upper body). **2.** Contract all the muscles in your body and pull yourself up, thinking about bringing your elbows to your sides and your chin over the bar so that it's parallel to the floor. Don't let your elbows flare out to the sides.

Lower yourself quickly but with control until you return to start position. Pause then repeat. There should be no bouncing out of the descent and no leg swing.

Chin-Up

Chin-ups are done the same way as a pull-up but with the exception of the palms facing in. These work the biceps more.

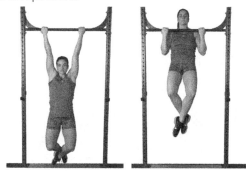

1. Hang from the bar with your hands in line with your shoulders or slightly wider and your palms facing you. Pack your shoulders in their sockets and allow your legs and elbows to be slightly bent (this keeps tension through the upper body). **2.** Contract all the muscles in your body and pull yourself up, thinking about bringing your elbows to your sides and your chin over the bar so that it's parallel to the floor. Don't let your elbows flare out to the sides.

Lower yourself quickly but with control until you return to start position. Pause then repeat. There should be no bouncing out of the descent and no leg swing.

Inverted Row

If pull-ups are too tough, work on inverted rows. The angle of your torso to the floor determines the difficulty of this movement. The closer to parallel you are, the harder the inverted row; the more upright you are, the easier it is. These can also be done using a suspension system such as TRX or Jungle Gym.

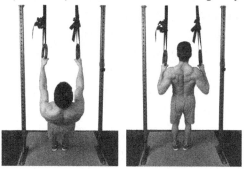

1. Set up a barbell on a squat rack so you can hang beneath it with your arms fully extended and torso parallel to the floor. Grab the bar with your hands about shoulder-width apart, palms facing away; this is basically a face-up plank position. **2.** Pull your chest to the bar while maintaining a rigid spine and squeezing your shoulder blades back. Keep your elbows in, close to your body.

Forearm Plank

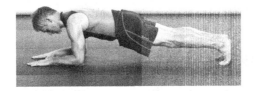

THE POSITION: Place your forearms on the floor parallel to each other; align your elbows under your shoulders. You may keep your palms face down on the floor or place the outer edges of your hands/fists on the floor. Extend your legs behind you like you would for a push-up, keeping your hips in the same plane as your shoulders. Squeeze your abs, glutes, hamstrings, quads, arms—everything but your neck—and hold that position. Make sure your back is flat; don't let your back sag or your hips go high or low.

VARIATIONS: To make the forearm plank more challenging, you can do a number of things:

- Use a resistance band around your mid-back, holding one end in each hand.

- Use a weight vest.

- Move the forearms forward so that your elbows are in front of your shoulders.

- Pull backward with your forearms while pulling down and forward with your toes. This should turn on your glutes, chest, and back much more than the standard plank.

High Plank

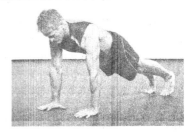

THE POSITION: Instead of working from your forearms, assume the top position of a push-up, placing your hands on the floor so that they're in line with your shoulders.

Super Plank

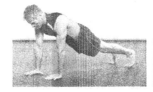 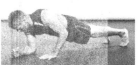

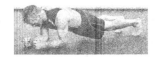

HOW LONG TO HOLD THE PLANK

There are different thoughts on how long to hold a plank. Some insist that you should be able to hold a forearm plank for at least 2 minutes, while others think that you're better off making the plank harder and holding for 10–20 seconds at most. I think you should mix it up and do both. That way you're working on core endurance (longer time) and also strength (heavier, harder variations, short duration).

With side planks, 90 seconds per side is considered minimally acceptable. You can wear a weight vest or use a resistance band around the hips to make it more challenging.

1. Start in a push-up position with your hands under your shoulders and your legs extended behind you.   **2.** Place one forearm on the floor so that the elbow is under that shoulder and the hand is straight out in front.   **3.** Now place the other forearm on the floor so that you're in a forearm plank.   **4.** Place one hand under that shoulder and start to straighten out that elbow.   **5.** As your torso starts to come up, lift the other forearm up and place that hand under the shoulder and finish straightening your elbows. You should be back in a push-up position.

Mix up the order you move the arms to keep it interesting. Don't slide your arms up and down or you'll get carpet burn. Pick up the hand and place the forearm down. It's a very distinct movement.

Side Plank

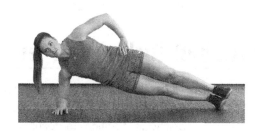

THE POSITION: Lie on the floor on your side, with your forearm on the floor so that your elbow is directly under your bottom shoulder. Stack your shoulders, hips, legs, and feet. Lift your torso, hips, and legs off the ground. Push your hips forward and make a straight line from the back of your head to your heels. Keep your entire body facing forward. Don't allow your torso or hips to rotate up or down. Hold, squeezing your abs and glutes hard.

Switch sides.

MODIFICATION: If you're rotating at the shoulders, torso, or hips (a sign of core weakness), position your back against a wall.

VARIATIONS: To make the side plank more challenging, lift your hips up and down but make sure you don't fold at the hips. You can also work on strengthening the abductors (the muscles that move the legs away from the midline) by raising the top leg while in the side plank position.

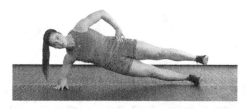

Side Plank with Hip Raise

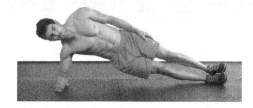

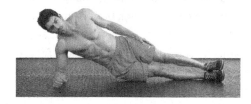

1. Lie on the floor on your side. Place your forearm on the floor so that your elbow is directly under the bottom shoulder. Stack your shoulders, hips, legs, and feet. Lift your torso, hips, and legs off the ground. Push your hips forward and make a straight line from the back of your head to your heels. Keep your entire body facing forward.   **2.** Now lower your hips, almost touching the floor. Don't let your body rotate or fold at the hips. You must still maintain a neutral spine.

Repeat the movement then switch sides.

Kettlebell Slingshot

This around-the-body pass is a very dynamic core stability exercise that should help *prevent* body rotation, so don't allow your body to move while performing this drill.

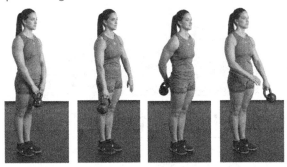

1. Stand with your feet together and hold a light bell with both hands in front of you, arms hanging down and elbows straight. Your left thumb and first two fingers should be holding the left corner of the handle while your right thumb and first two fingers hold the right corner, both palms facing the rear. **2.** Release the bell from one hand and move both arms behind you, one to each side. As you do the Slingshot, your hands will always face the rear. **3–4.** Without moving your torso, bending at your ribs or twisting, use your free hand to grab the handle by the open corner and release the other hand. Keep your abs, glutes, and lower back locked together throughout the movement to prevent your torso from bending or turning. **5.** Bring both arms back to the front and transfer the bell to the other hand.

Continue passing the bell around your body, then switch directions.

Some things to keep in mind:

- The torso should not bend or rotate in any manner.
- Any movement of the body comes through the feet and ankles and is an automatic

response to counterbalance the body against the weight. If you're using a moderately heavy bell, this will probably happen. If you're using a light bell, it might not unless you're moving it very fast.

- Don't lift the bell with the arms, especially when the bell is passing in front of the body. This can cause some elbow problems.
- Make sure there's nothing that can be damaged or hurt if you miss the transition from one hand to the other. It's normal at first to miss and drop the bell. If you do, it will fly away from you so make sure you have adequate clearance and there are no kids or pets nearby.
- The transition from one hand to the other must occur when your hands are in the center line of the body. If the transfer occurs off to one side, you'll rotate your torso that way.

Kettlebell Turkish Get-Up

The Turkish Get-Up, or TGU, is a whole-body exercise that requires a tremendous amount of shoulder stability and mobility. In addition to focusing on your shoulders, abs, and hips, it improves your glute strength and hip mobility, works the lunge pattern, and a lot more. Going light and slow is considerably harder than it looks. Going heavy requires a lot more body awareness and control than what you'd ever imagine. We'll move through the TGU movements quickly here but if you want more details, check out my other Ulysses Press book *The Ultimate Kettlebell Workbook*, where the TGU is broken down into its component parts.

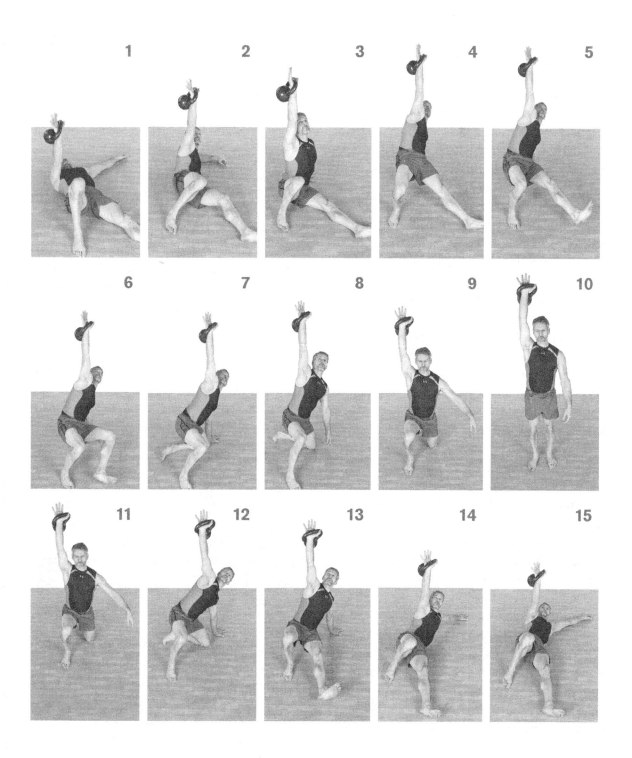

1. Lie flat on your back and press a bell with your right arm. Bend your right knee to about 45 degrees with the foot flat on the floor; your left leg remains straight. Your left arm is on the floor and out to the side at shoulder level, while your right arm is locked and vertical. **2–3.** Driving with your right foot, roll from your upper left arm to your elbow and forearm so that you end up with your left palm flat on the floor supporting you and almost directly under your shoulder; your torso should be upright. Your right knee is still bent and pointing up, while your left leg is straight. **4–5.** Driving your right heel into the floor, lift your butt as high as you can into a bridge position. Keep your hips facing the ceiling. At the same time, drive your left shoulder into the floor by pushing the hand hard against the floor. Let your left leg rotate from the hip so that the outside edge of the foot is on the floor. **6–8.** Bring your left leg under you, bending the knee and placing it just in front of your left hand. Your right shin is now close to vertical and your right foot is flat on the floor. **9.** Swing your lower left leg out from under you and pivot on your knee so that your left foot is directly behind you; your torso should come up at the same time. You're now in a half kneeling position. **10.** Flip onto the ball of your left foot and drive from the heel of the front foot and the ball of the back foot to a standing position. As you stand, bring your left foot forward next to your right foot. **11.** To return to the floor, step back with your left foot as in a back lunge and place your left knee gently on the floor. **12.** Flip your left foot so that the top of the foot is on the floor. Rotating at the hip, swing your lower left leg under you so that your toes point to the right. At the same time, push your hips to the right and place your left hand on the floor by the left knee, driving your shoulder down away from your ear. Your right knee is bent and your shin is almost vertical with your right foot, which is flat on the floor. **13.** Support yourself on your left hand and flat right foot. Lift your hips and

shoot your left leg out from under you, extending your knee and letting the outside of the foot rest on the floor. **14–15.** Slowly slide your left arm out from under you toward the left rear. Let your forearm then your upper arm roll to the floor. Your left side then comes into contact with the floor. Roll onto your back and into start position.

From here, you have three options: 1. Bring the bell down to the floor, drag it to the other side, and do a rep on the left. 2. Leave your right arm extended and do another rep on the right. 3. Or re-press the bell on the right and repeat the get-up. Option 1 is usually used when going heavy, option 2 for when you're lifting light, option 3 for moderate weight.

Carioca

This is a great footwork drill as well as fantastic hip opener. For clarity we'll be moving to the right. You may also hold your arms out to the sides, which can help you determine if your torso is turning (it shouldn't be).

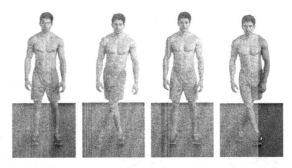

1. Stand with your feet about shoulder-width apart. **2.** Step with your left foot so that it crosses in front of your right. **3.** Step out with your right foot to shoulder width. **4.** Now step your left foot behind your right foot. As you step, pivot your hip sharply to the left. **5.** Step out with your right back to shoulder width, with hips facing straight ahead. **6.** Step with your left foot in front of your right again. **7.** Step out to shoulder width with your right.   **8.** Step behind with your left foot, pivoting your hips to the right.

Go 20 yards or until you run out of room, then reverse the movement and get back to your starting point.

Fast Feet Drill

Use a sturdy low box or aerobic step and make sure it can't slide. You'll be moving across the narrow part of the box or step. If your box is too wide, this won't work very well. We'll start by moving to the left. Over time this will dramatically improve your foot work.

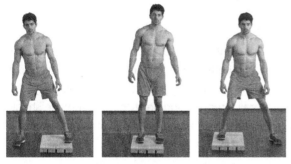

1. Stand next to the step with your body facing the same direction as the step. Pick up your left foot and place it on the far side of the step.   **2.** Quickly bring your other foot onto the step.   **3.** Step off to the left with your left foot and immediately follow with your right foot. Both feet are on the floor and the step is on your right side.   **4.** Quickly step your right foot to the right side of the step and immediately follow with your left.   **5.** Step off to the right with your right foot and follow with your left. You're back at start position.

Burpee

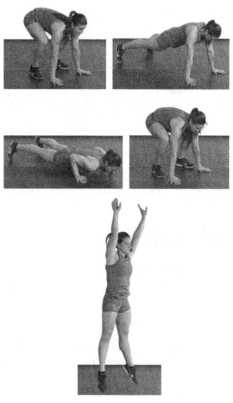

1. Stand with your feet shoulder-width apart. **2.** Squat down deeply and put your hands on the floor inside your feet.   **3–4.** Kick both feet back so that you're in a solid push-up/high plank position. Try to keep your hips low.   **5.** Do a push-up.   **6.** Bring both knees back under you and shift from the balls of your feet to a flat foot position and stand—or, better yet, jump.

VARIATION: For a more challenging version, land in the bottom of a push-up position instead of the top for steps 3–5. The only difference is you bend your elbows as your hands touch the floor, allowing your shoulders and pecs to absorb the fall. If you have shoulder problems don't do this variation.

If you're unable to squat deeply and place your hands on the floor, you need to work on your hip mobility by doing Bootstrappers (page 154).

Mountain Climber

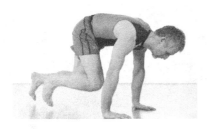

1. Assume a high plank with one knee tucked under you. You'll be supporting your weight with your upper body throughout the movement. Keep your elbows locked and hands shoulder-width apart.

2. Switch feet by quickly driving the tucked knee back and pulling the other knee under you. Your feet should not slide along the floor. The only time your feet touch the floor is the split second when one knee is up under you and the other leg is fully extended. As soon as you hit that position, move right through it and keep going. You shouldn't kick your feet up toward your butt. If you do, use a pair of furniture sliders under your feet when performing mountain climbers; this will force you to do the move correctly.

CRAWLING

Crawling exercises are very challenging bodyweight movements that help create and maintain a strong core and mobile hips; they can also help your shoulder blades function better. Crawling duplicates the cross-body movement pattern that you use when walking or running and forces your body to respond reflexively. This fundamental movement pattern teaches coordination and overall strength, and pretty much everyone should add crawling to their workouts, whether as a warm-up, part of the main training session, or at the end as a finisher. However, avoid these movements if you have shoulder pain when doing push-ups.

Bear Crawl

Crawling builds core strength and upper-body strength, and gets the upper back to stabilize the shoulders while the body moves around them. This fundamental movement is extremely beneficial. Unless you have a severe shoulder issue, almost everyone should try some form of crawling. You may find it tough at first but you should be able to work up to it. The bear crawl starts like the Quad Press (page 153) but you may allow your hips to come up a little.

1. Start on your hands and knees, with your hands a little wider than your shoulders, your knees slightly behind your hips, and your feet as wide as your hands.   **2.** Move one arm and the opposite leg forward.   **3.** Shift your weight slightly then move the other arm and leg.

Ideally the hand and opposite foot move at the same time rather than hand, foot, then foot. Make sure you aren't allowing your hips to travel sideways; there should be no swaying.

Try to go 2 minutes.

VARIATION: You can do the bear crawl backward. As you get better, move the hand and opposite foot at the same time instead of one at a time.

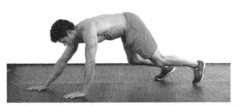

Spiderman Crawl

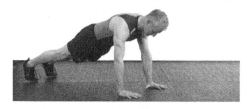

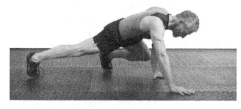

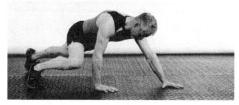

1. Start in push-up plank position. **2.** Move your right hand forward and place it on the floor. As the hand plants, lower yourself down by bending both elbows. At the same time, bring your left knee up toward your left elbow. Your inner thigh should be parallel to the floor. **3.** Push up and move your left hand forward, straighten your bent leg, plant your hand, and bring your right leg up with the inner thigh parallel to the floor. Don't rotate your pelvis—even though your hips are moving to the sides, they're still parallel to the floor.

VARIATION: As you get better, move the hand and opposite foot at the same time.

Spiderman Push-Up & Crawl

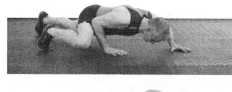

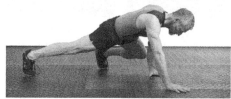

This exercise gets its name because you look like Spiderman when he scales a building. If you can't do a Spiderman Push-Up (page 153), don't worry about the crawl. This killer ab movement will improve your hip mobility as well.

1. Assume a push-up plank position. **2.** As you slowly lower down, bring your right knee up toward your right elbow and rotate that hip so that your inner thigh is just off the floor. **3.** As you push up, return the leg to its starting position. **4.** On the next rep, bring your other knee up.

Alternate legs each rep.

SKIPPING

Skipping is another fundamental movement pattern that teaches the opposite hand-leg pattern. Your body is a big X, with the center of your torso as the center of the X. Your right upper body and left lower body work together, as do the left upper and right lower bodies. The left hemisphere controls the right side and the right hemisphere controls the left side. This explains why you can have an injured right hip and later develop problems in your left shoulder; the muscles and fascia crisscross your body through the center of the X.

Marching in Place

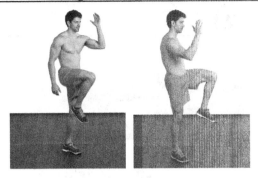

1. Stand with your feet hip-width apart and arms hanging by your sides. **2.** Raise your right knee until your thigh is parallel to the floor or higher, but don't overdo it—keep your spine neutral. At the same time your knee comes up, raise your left arm while bending at the elbow. Your left hand should be shoulder height. **3.** Lower your leg and arm at the same time. **4.** Lift your left knee up to parallel and your right hand up to about shoulder height, bending the elbow. **5.** Lower your arm and leg.

Walking with Knee and Arm Raise

Once you can do Marching in Place without hiking a hip or bending forward, try adding locomotion.

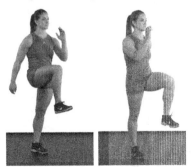

1. Start as you did with the marching in place and then bring your right knee and left arm up. **2.** Lower

your arm and leg but place your right foot forward as though you took a normal step. Shift your weight to your right foot and bring your left knee and right arm up. **3.** Lower your left and step forward onto it while lowering your right arm. **4.** Shift your weight to the left and bring your right knee and left arm up again.

Keep walking while raising the arm and leg.

Skipping Forward

1. Stand with your arms by your sides. **2.** Lift your right knee as high as possible and raise your left arm, bending the elbow until your hand is in front of your shoulder. As your right knee and left arm come up, rise up onto the ball of your left foot and propel yourself forward a little. **3.** Land on your right foot and lower your left hand. **4.** Hop forward a little, driving from your right foot, and bring your left knee and right arm up to skip on the other side.

Repeat.

Side Shuffle

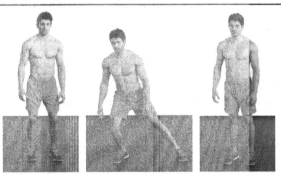

1. Stand with your feet hip-width apart, knees slightly bent, and hips back. **2.** Lift and turn your right foot toward the right and plant your heel. **3.** Pull yourself to the right by digging in with your right heel and pulling with your right leg rather than stepping with your left. You may feel this in your right inner thigh. Pick up your left foot but don't drag it on the floor.

Go 10–20 yards then do the same using your left foot to start.

Sprinting

Run really, really fast, pumping the arms. The movement is similar to skipping without the hop.

Ok, so there's more to it than that, but there are plenty of resources to teach you proper sprint mechanics. As long as you don't have any hip or knee issues, just run. If you had a tough time with the self-assessments for the lunge, hurdle step, or active straight-leg raise, you shouldn't run.

Your time or distance should be as far as you can go without slowing down. If you aren't maintaining top speed, you aren't sprinting. Typically 20 seconds will be all you can do, but at the beginning stages it will be more like 5–10 seconds. This would translate into 10–20 yards. When you consider the top sprinters run 100 meters in slightly under 10 seconds, you'll soon realize that you'll only be able to sustain all-out effort for a very brief burst.

Rest at least 2 minutes between sprints to ensure full recovery.

HEAVY ROPE TRAINING

Sometimes called battling ropes, the heavy ropes you'll need are 30 feet or longer and 1.5- to 2-inches in diameter. You'll also need an anchor of some sort to loop the rope through or around. A round post works well, but it must be smooth or the rope will wear out quickly. You'll move your arms and body to create waves in the rope. This sounds pretty basic but, trust me, it's a tough conditioning exercise.

Double Wave

The most basic pattern is the double wave, where both arms move up and down simultaneously while your hips move up and down. By using your hips in addition to your arms, you turn the movement into a full-body exercise. You can make big waves and slow down or you can create short waves and go fast. The former trains power, the latter speed and, depending on how long you go, endurance.

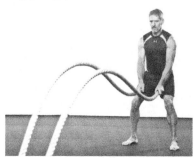

1. Stand facing the anchor with one end of the rope in each hand, feet shoulder-width apart, hands at hip height, elbows bent, and knees slightly bent. Your back should be neutral. The position is close to the hang position for the clean. **2–3.** Sink down with your hips, bending your knees a little more, and stand up quickly, raising your forearms up and flexing your wrists. **4.** Quickly drop down and let your forearms and wrists drop as well. Keep your elbows close to your sides. **5.** Rapidly reverse directions up and down, your arms moving with your legs. It's a pumping action.

How high your hands come up determines how big the wave and how hard you slam the ropes down.

SHORT-WAVE VARIATION: To train for speed, keep your elbows close to your lower ribs instead of hip height and move primarily from your wrists with some elbow flexion. Extend your hips and knees as you flex your elbows, then quickly reverse the movement by flexing your hips, knees, elbows, and wrists. This should be a short, quick movement with very little power.

Alternating Waves

The only difference between alternating waves and double waves is that your arms move opposite each other. One moves up while the other moves down. This will cause your hips to rotate from side to side.

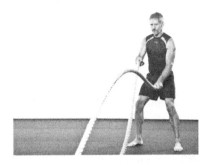

1. Start the same as the Double Wave (page 165). **2.** Move one arm up and the other down in unison, with pumping action from the legs. There'll be more of a sideways movement of the hips rather than straight up and down. Make sure you're moving

through your wrists—don't keep them locked in. The hand/arm movement is a drumming pattern.

In/Out Waves

In this tough variation, you must learn to keep your wrists relaxed or the rope won't move well. Try to alternate the top hand each rep.

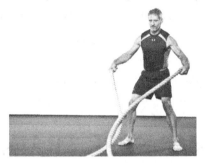

1. Start the same as the Double Wave (page 165). **2.** Separate your arms to your sides as you straighten your knees. **3.** Quickly reverse your movement, bending your knees and bringing your arms in so that your wrists cross at your navel. While crossed, your hands shouldn't be any more than chest-width apart. **4.** Rapidly reverse, moving your hands back out to the sides. Keep your elbows in to prevent your hands from going too far apart.

CARRIES

Carries are exactly what the name implies—you'll be carrying a weight that you move and hold in different positions as you walk. You can use a barbell or a kettlebell for all of these and a dumbbell for most of them. If you have access to a sandbag, you can use that, too.

Farmer's Walk

You can go long and light or short and heavy. This move is brutal if you chose to go heavy and long! Using barbells for this move is very tough; the wide load makes it hard to find the balance point and harder to maintain it. They actually make bars with handles specifically to work this movement for those who do strongman training and competitions.

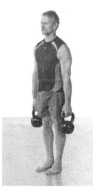

1. Pick up a weight in each hand, keeping each arm hanging straight down by your side. **2.** Stand tall, keep your shoulders in their sockets, and walk. Make sure not to lean forward—keep your chest up and shoulders back at all times. Make sure you aren't letting the weight pull your shoulders out of their sockets; engage all the muscles in your arms, shoulders, and back.

ONE-ARM VARIATION (SUITCASE CARRY): The one-arm variation works the obliques on the side opposite the weight and your grip, arm, shoulders, and traps on the same side as the weight.

Rack Walk

This can be done with 1 or 2 kettlebells. One-arm rack walks work the body similar to the Farmer's Walk but, with the bell on your chest, you have to learn to breathe around them. These hit the core, shoulder, and upper back hard. Go heavy and long for best results.

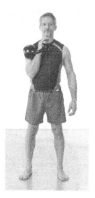

1. Hold the bell(s) in the kettlebell rack position with your elbow bent and your entire arm resting against your body. **2.** Walk.

Waiter's Walk

With kettlebells you can either hold the handle in your palm and the bell on the outside of your forearm, or you can hold the ball portion of the bell in your palm with your palm facing up. Go light—these are very deceptively hard. If you have shoulder mobility issues, don't do doubles.

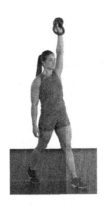

1. Hold 1 or 2 kettlebells overhead. Keep your elbows locked.   **2.** Walk. You'll feel like a waiter carrying a tray.

Bottom's-Up Walk

These can only be done with a kettlebell. Go light; this requires really strong hands to keep the bell from falling.

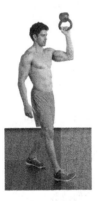

1. Hold 1 or 2 kettlebells by the center of the handle with the bottom of the bell facing up (holding the corner of the handle is cheating). Your elbow can be down like in the rack walk, or you can keep your upper arm parallel to the floor, which is quite a bit harder.   **2.** Walk.

Once you've gotten the hang of those mix things up a bit.

- Option 1: Farmer's Walk: light on one side, heavy on the other. Switch halfway.

- Option 2: Farmer's Walk on one side, Waiter's Walk on the other. Switch halfway.

- Option 3: Farmer's Walk on one side, Rack Walk or Bottom's-Up Walk on the other. Switch halfway.

Goblet Carry

This can be done with a kettlebell or dumbbell. Regardless, it will fry your biceps.

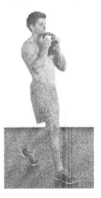

1. Like in the Goblet Squat (page 146), hold a kettlebell with both hands by its "horns" at sternum level. The bell will be close to your body but not touching, and your elbows should be down.
2. Start walking.

PART 5
EXERCISE FIXES

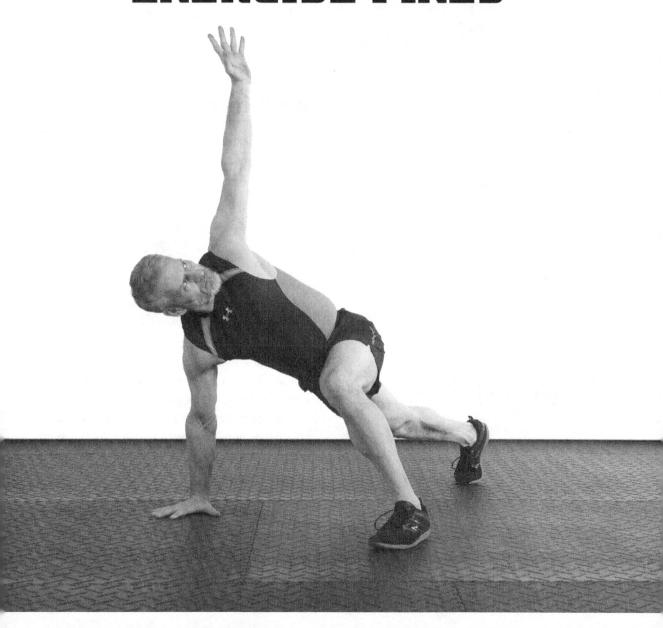

Quad Extension Rotation

Make sure you're rotating and not bending your spine—the goal is to open your upper back and chest. There should be no movement below your mid-back.

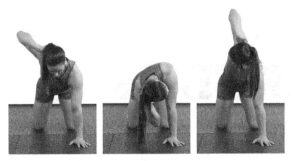

1. Get on all fours with your thighs and arms vertical and hands shoulder-width apart. Your knees are directly under your hips. Keeping a neutral spine, lift your right hand behind your head, resting your palm on the back of your neck, elbow pointing to the side. Actively drive your left arm into the floor to support your bodyweight; don't sink into your shoulder.   **2.** Inhale then exhale as you slowly rotate your torso downward and inward through your upper back and neck to bring your right elbow between your left arm and thigh.   **3.** Inhale then exhale as you slowly reverse the rotation, bringing your right elbow up until it's pointing to the ceiling. Make sure your head moves with your elbow.

Repeat 4 more times then switch sides.

Forearm Wall Slide

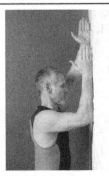

1. Face a wall, standing 6–12 inches away. Bend your elbows and place your forearms on the wall, palms facing each other; lean so that your forearms bear some of your weight. Your elbows should be level with your shoulders. Inhale.   **2.** Engaging your core to keep your body stationary, exhale as you slowly slide one forearm straight up with control, maintaining contact with the wall. Try to straighten your elbow; if you can't, don't force it. Try to prevent any torso rotation toward the side you're working.   **3.** At the top, briefly inhale then exhale and slowly slide that arm back down with control to the start position.

Switch sides. Do 10–12 reps per arm.

Back-to-Wall Arm Slide

If you're locked up in the upper back, this will be *very* tough and you may experience a cramp in the muscles between your shoulder blades.

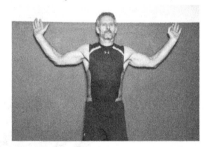

1. Stand with your head and back against a wall. Move your feet away from the wall as needed to get your back in the proper position.   **2.** Bend your elbows to about 90 degrees and rotate your arms upward so that your forearms are on the wall with your hands about level with your shoulders, palms facing forward.   **3.** Inhale then exhale as you slide both arms up the wall and outward a little until you can no longer keep your forearms on the wall. Pause.   **4.** Inhale then exhale as you slide your arms back to the start position.

Do 12–15 reps.

VARIATION: This can also be done while lying on the floor with your knees bent. Place your arms on the floor with your hands at about shoulder level, palms up. Inhale then exhale as you slide both arms up and out until your forearms or hands come off the floor. Pause. Inhale then exhale as you slide both arms back to the start position.

Band-Assisted Pec Stretch

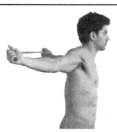

1. Stand holding a resistance band in both hands in front of your thighs, palms facing backward and elbows straight with a little slack.   **2.** Raise your arms behind you with your hands about shoulder-width apart. The band will be behind your head. The tension in the band should pull your hands farther back. Exhale to relax into the stretch. Hold for 10 seconds or until it gets uncomfortable.   **3.** Inhale and bring your hands forward to release the stretch.   **4.** Exhale and re-engage the stretch, letting the band pull your hands farther back.

Do this 5–10 times.

Spiderman with Rotation

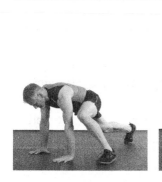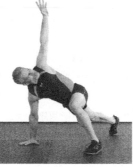

1. Assume a High Plank (page 182). Inhale then exhale as you bring your left foot forward and outside your left hand. Try to get it as close to your hand as possible while keeping it pointed forward and your heel down.   **2.** Inhale then exhale as you rotate your upper body toward your left leg so that your left arm goes overhead. Turn your head to follow your hand with your eyes.   **3.** Inhale and bring your hand back to the floor.

Return to a high plank and repeat on the other side.

Do a total of 20 reps, alternating sides.

Halo

These can be done from standing or the half-kneeling or tall-kneeling positions. Half kneeling is more challenging than standing in terms of body stability. This is a fluid, controlled exercise—don't rush the circular movement.

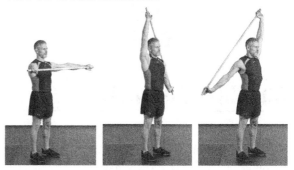

1. Hold a band, PVC pipe, or broomstick with your hands shoulder-width apart at chest level. If you're using a band, keep a little tension in it.   **2.** Keeping both elbows straight, bring your right arm to the left and let your left hand drop to your left hip. Inhale.   **3.** As your right hand moves to the left, let your right arm pass over your head as you bring it behind you. At the same time, bring your left arm up so that it goes overhead and then to the front near your right shoulder. You should be the opposite of Step 2.

Continue the movement, bringing your right arm up as your left arm goes down to the left.

Exhale as you return to start position.

Do 5 times then reverse the movement.

KETTLEBELL VARIATION: **1.** Hold the kettlebell in both hands with the handle facing down and your elbows bent. The bell is close to your chest but not touching. **2.** Inhaling, move the bell to the left, rotating your arms so that your right forearm goes overhead, brushing your hair (if you have any!). Keep the bell at neck level as the bell moves behind you. **3.** Continue the movement by bringing the bell to the right, allowing your left forearm to brush your hair. Exhale as you return to start position.

Do 10 times then change directions.

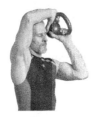

Shoulder Dislocate

This opens the shoulders, chest, and back; over time you should be able to get your hands fairly close together. If you can't do the full range of motion (from the hips in front to the glutes in back), widen your grip. If it's too easy, bring your hands in.

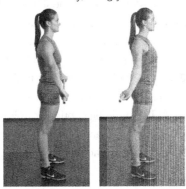

1. With your arms hanging down and elbows straight, take an end of a band, PVC pipe, or towel in each hand. **2.** Keeping your elbows straight, raise your arms overhead and behind you until the band, PVC pipe, or towel is touching your butt. As your arms go behind you, relax your grip a little so that your hands can move around the band, PVC pipe, or towel. **3.** Keeping your arms straight, bring the band, PVC pipe, or towel back to the front.

Do 10 reps.

Side-Lying Windmill

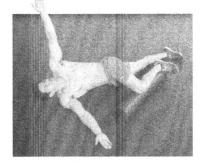

1. Lie on your side, legs extended, with a foam roller in front of you parallel to your body. Place your top leg's knee, shin, and foot on the roller with your hip and knee bent 90 degrees. Your hips should be pointing forward, not toward the floor or up. Extend both arms directly from your shoulders, arms together, elbows straight. **2.** Extend the top shoulder by reaching forward with the arm. Don't allow your hips to shift. Inhale then exhale as you sweep your top arm in a semicircle behind you, keeping your elbow straight and your hand as close to the floor as possible. If you feel the foam roller moving, you're moving from your lower back instead of your upper back. **3.** Inhale when the top arm is directly opposite the bottom arm, then exhale and bring the arm over the body and back to start position. Don't hold your breath.

Do 5 reps then switch sides.

Bretzel

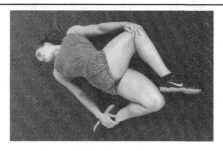

THE POSITION: Lie on your side with your knees bent. Bring your bottom leg behind you and grab the foot with the opposite hand. If you can't reach it, use a yoga strap or resistance band. Try to keep the side of the foot on the floor. Place the foot of the top leg against the front of the bottom leg. Use the opposite hand to hold the knee on the floor. Inhale then exhale and roll the top shoulder and head toward the floor behind you. Don't let the front knee come off the floor. Hold the exhale for a few seconds, inhale, exhale again, and try to get the shoulder closer to the floor. Don't let the knee on the front leg come off the floor.

Repeat for 30 seconds then switch sides. You'll most likely find one side comes much closer to the floor than the other.

Lat Stretch with Band

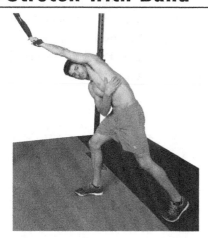

THE POSITION: Attach a heavy/thick resistance band to a pull-up bar or squat rack about 1 foot over your head. Don't use a therapy band for this—it will break! Place your right wrist inside the band then grasp the band in your right hand with your hand facing across your body. Step back and behind yourself with your right foot. Make sure there's tension in the band; if there isn't, step back more. Rotate your torso to the right, maintaining neutral spine. Don't round or overly extend your lower back. Place your left hand on the right side of your chest or lats. Sink back into your right hip until you feel a stretch through your lat. Don't let your right arm rotate; your palm should always face across your body.

Move in and out of this for about 1 minute by relaxing then pulling against the band. Switch sides.

Arm Bar

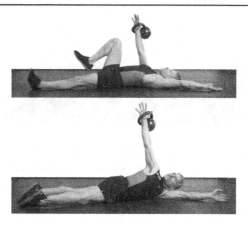

1. Lie face-up on the floor with your legs extended. With your right hand press a kettlebell until your arm is vertical. It MUST remain vertical throughout this movement or you'll lose control.   **2.** Bend your right knee and place your left arm alongside your head on the floor.   **3.** Pick up your right foot and bring the knee across your body so that you start to roll over.   **4.** Keeping your eyes on the bell as you roll, cross your right knee over your left. Begin to straighten your right knee and place your right foot near your left foot. At this point you should be almost facedown with your kettlebell arm still vertical and your head looking toward the bell. Hold for 3–5 seconds.

Reverse the movement to return to start position.

Do 3–5 reps then bring the bell down and put it on the floor. Switch sides by either turning around or by dragging the bell on floor and around your head (*not* across your body).

Standing Knee-to-Wall Ankle Mobility

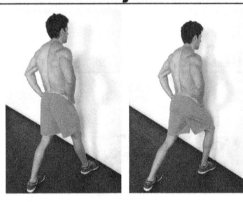

1. Stand in front of a wall with your right foot about 5 inches from the wall and your left foot behind you.   **2.** Inhale then exhale as you drive your right knee toward the wall, keeping your foot flat on the floor. If you can touch the wall, move your right foot back another inch. You should feel a stretch in your calf. Don't worry about the back leg.   **3.** Hold the position for a few seconds then inhale as you straighten the knee back to start position.

Do 10 reps then switch sides.

Toe Pull 1

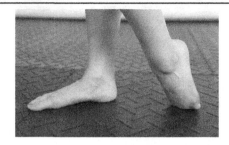

1. Stand barefoot with your left foot behind you and the top of the foot on the floor.   **2.** Pull your left foot gently downward and forward into the floor without moving the foot.   **3.** Rotate your foot around the point of contact while maintaining the "pull."

Do 10 reps then switch sides.

Toe Pull 2

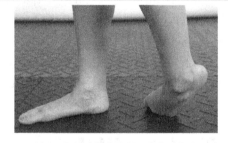

1. Stand barefoot with your left foot behind you and the top outside part of the foot on the floor. **2.** Pull downward and forward with your left foot.   **3.** Rotate your foot around the point of contact while maintaining the "pull."

Do 10 reps then switch sides.

Calf Stretch

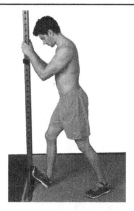

1. Stand in a staggered stance facing a wall with your right leg forward. **2.** Place the ball of your right foot on the wall and the heel on the floor. Your right knee should be lined up with your hip and the middle toe, while your left leg is behind you with the left foot and knee aligned with your left hip. **3.** Moving through your hips, drive your right knee toward the wall so your torso leans into it. You should feel a stretch in your right calf. Hold the stretch for a few seconds then release.

Do 10 reps then switch sides.

Lower Legs Roller Release

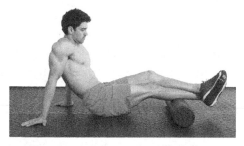

1. Sit on the floor with your legs straight and one leg crossed over the other. Place your crossed legs on a horizontal foam roller, finding the most uncomfortable spot. Stay relaxed and breathe while visualizing the muscles relaxing.

MASSAGE STICK VARIATION: Get on one knee. In a slow and controlled manner, roll the stick up and down the outside of the lower leg, the inside on the shin bone, the back of the lower leg, and down into the Achilles tendon. Relax when you find tender areas.

Hip Rock Back

Keep this movement slow and deliberate and learn to feel what your hips are doing. It's helpful to have someone place a PVC pipe or broomstick on your back so that the back of your head, between your shoulder blades and the base of your spine, are all in contact with the stick. There should be a slight gap between your lower back and the stick. As you rock back, stop when the stick changes contact points or you feel your tailbone rounding under. Use your abs to control your pelvis but it shouldn't be a hard effort.

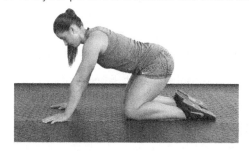

1. Get on all fours, hands shoulder-width apart, arms and thighs vertical, and knees under your hips. **2.** Keeping your spine neutral, inhale then exhale as you push away from the ground with your arms. Maintaining neutral spine, sit back into your hips as far as possible until your tailbone rolls under. Pause for 2 seconds. **3.** Inhale and rock forward.

Do 10 reps.

Leg-Abducted Rock Back

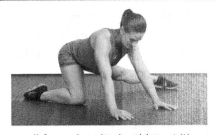

1. Get on all fours, hands shoulder-width apart, arms and thighs vertical, and knees under your hips. Keeping your foot flat on the floor and toes pointing forward, extend your left leg directly to the side so that the middle of the foot is straight out from the left knee. Make sure your left leg is straight.   **2.** Keeping your spine neutral, inhale then exhale as you push away from the ground with your arms. Maintaining neutral spine, rock back into your hips. Use a stick on your back as described in Hip Rock Back (page 175) to check your alignment. You may feel a stretch in the inner thigh of the extended leg. Pause for 2 seconds.   **3.** Inhale and rock forward.

Do 10–12 reps then switch sides.

Face-the-Wall Squat

The goal of this exercise is to teach you to squat while keeping your torso relatively upright and not allowing it to fold over, which is an indication of weak abs. This also teaches you to pull your hips down but not back.

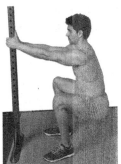

1. Stand facing a wall with your feet about 6 inches away. Lift your arms to shoulder height, palms facing the wall.   **2.** Inhale then exhale as you sit down and back into your hips without letting any part of your body touch the wall. Go as deep as you can without falling backward.   **3.** Inhale and return to starting position.

If you can't do this from the 6-inch distance, move back about an inch.

Do 10 reps.

Leg Lowering 1

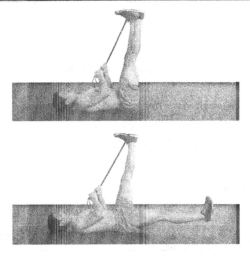

1. Lie on your back and loop a strap around your left foot. Extend both legs straight up to the ceiling. The toes of both feet should be pulled back toward your shins (dorsiflexion), which helps to keep the knees straight.   **2.** Inhale through your nose then exhale hard through your mouth (like you're blowing up a balloon) while lowering your right leg toward the floor without touching the floor. Your breathing controls the speed of the leg going down; it should be about a 6 count. Keep your right leg stationary in the vertical position. Don't arch your back.   **3.** Once the exhale is complete and your foot is almost touching the floor, hold the exhale for a 3 count. **4.** Inhale for a 3 count to bring your right leg back up, keeping the knee straight throughout the movement. No other part of your body should move.

Do 10 reps then switch sides.

Leg Lowering 2

Once you can do Leg Lowering 1 with your strapped leg close to vertical, it's time to do the move without the strap.

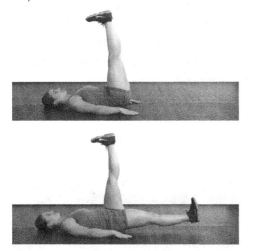

1. Lie on your back and raise both legs as close to vertical as you can while keeping your knees straight. Pull the toes of both feet up toward your shins. **2.** Inhale through your nose then exhale hard through your mouth while lowering your left leg toward the floor without touching the floor. Your breathing controls the speed of the leg going down; it should be about a 6 count. Keep your right leg stationary in the vertical position. Don't arch your back. **3.** Once the exhale is complete and your foot is almost touching the floor, hold the exhale for a 3 count. **4.** Inhale for a 3 count to bring your left leg back up, keeping the knee straight throughout the movement. No other part of your body should move.

Do 10 reps then switch sides.

One-Leg Glute Bridge

If during the ASLR self-assessment (page 34) one side was better than the other, you'll need to strengthen the weaker side with this exercise.

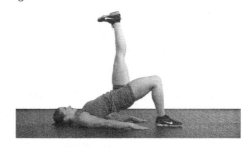

1. Lie on your back and brace your abs a little to push your lower back into the floor. Bend the knee on the weak side and place the foot flat on the floor. Keeping your back neutral at all times, raise the strong-side leg straight up with the knee straight. **2.** Inhale through your nose then exhale hard through your mouth. While exhaling for a 6 count, squeeze your glutes and lift your hips off the floor, moving with the speed of the exhale. Don't hyperextend (arch) your back or rotate your pelvis. Make sure you hips remain level while performing this exercise. Pause at the top and hold the exhale for a 3 count. **3.** Inhale through your nose for a 3 count while lowering your hips to the floor. Focus on glute activation. If you feel this anywhere but your glutes, you're lifting with your leg instead of your hips. Adjust your movement.

Do 10 reps on your weak side. Don't do the strong side for now—you need to strengthen the weak side so it catches up to the stronger side.

VARIATION: Once this move becomes easy, you can add weight by holding a dumbbell or kettlebell on the hip of the working side.

Dead Bug (Bent Knees)

The Dead Bug works your core control and your brain by forcing you to learn to move your arms and legs independently while maintaining a neutral spine. There are several variations; in this book we focus on bent-knee and opposite-arm pattern and the more challenging straight-leg and opposite-arm versions. If you can't keep your knees straight while lying on your back with your legs vertical, do the Dead Bug bent-knee version plus Leg Lowering 1 (page 176).

In this bent-knee variation, we incorporate cross-body movement patterns that happen when you walk or run, among other things. This version is difficult to do correctly because you must keep your lower back on the floor and your body stationary while your arm and opposite leg move.

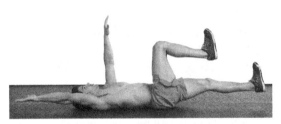

1. Lie on your back with your arms extended to the ceiling and both legs lifted with your knees bent 90 degrees, thighs vertical, and toes pulled back toward your shins. **2.** Inhale through your nose then exhale hard through your mouth for a 6 count while lowering one arm back toward the floor above your head and simultaneously extending the opposite leg out and down so that your heel is slightly off the floor. Pause at the bottom for a 3 count, holding your exhale. **3.** Inhale through your nose for a 3 count while returning the arm and leg back to start position. Again, nothing else should

move at any time except the working arm and the opposite leg.

Don't start the next rep until you're completely back to start position.

Perform 20 reps total, alternating the arm/leg pair each rep.

Dead Bug (Straight Legs)

This version should only be done if you can keep your knees straight as in Leg Lowering 2 (page 177). The straight legs make it even tougher to maintain your core and back due to the extended leverage involved. If you can't keep your knees straight, revert to the bent-knee variation.

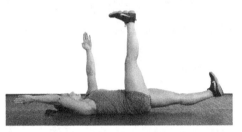

1. Lie on your back with your arms and legs extended to the ceiling, toes pulled back to your shins on both legs. **2.** Inhale through your nose then exhale hard through your mouth for a 6 count while lowering one arm back toward the floor above your head and the opposite leg down toward the floor with your heel leading the way. Don't let your heel touch the floor. Pause at the bottom for a 3 count, holding your exhale. **3.** Inhale through your nose for a 3 count while returning the arm and opposite leg back to start position.

Perform 20 reps total, alternating the arm/leg pair each rep.

Glute Bridge

You should feel this only in your butt. If you feel your hamstrings, you're pushing with your feet, not lifting your hips. Don't arch your lower back; if you start to feel it there after a few reps, you're most likely arching. Use your abs to control your back and pelvic position.

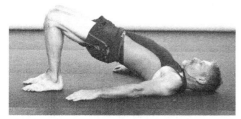

1. Lie flat on your back with your knees bent and the back of your head on the floor, chin tucked slightly.   **2.** Inhale then exhale through your mouth for a 6 count as you squeeze your glutes and forcefully lift your hips off the ground. Pause at the top for a 3 count, holding the exhale.   **3.** Inhale through your nose for a 3 count while lowering your hips back to the floor.

Do 10 reps.

ADVANCED VARIATION: Once the unweighted glute bridge is no longer challenging, it's time to add some weight. Place a sandbag, kettlebell, or dumbbell across your lower abs. You can even use heavy chains. Regardless of the type of resistance, it should be relatively heavy—your glutes are big and strong (or at least they should be). Do 10 reps.

Barbell Hip Thruster

This is a fantastic exercise to safely strengthen your hips, butt, and core—not your quads—so you'll really feel this in your glutes! Most people can move a lot of weight using this exercise. You'll need a padded bench that won't slide. If the bench moves during the exercise, you'll get seriously injured! Women should start with 95 pounds and men with 135 to get the feel of the movement. I'd expect most of you will be able to go quite a bit heavier—185 for women and probably 250 pounds or more for most guys, especially if you deadlift a lot.

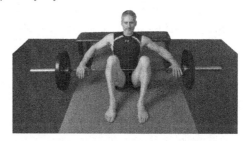

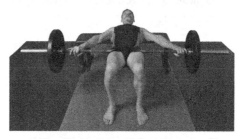

1. Load a barbell with bumper plates that are the same diameter as a regular 45-pound plate. Pad the bar with an Airex pad or yoga mat as the weight of the bar across your hips can be painful. Set up a padded bench horizontally against a wall or squat rack, making sure it can't slide out from under you. Sit on the floor in front of the bench with your shoulder blades resting against the side of the bench. Position the bar over your hips, just above groin level, then hold it with your hands (palms down).   **2.** Bend your knees and place your feet flat on the floor. Your feet and knees should be directly in line with your hips or you might strain your knees. At this point the bar should be in contact with your hips.   **3.** Inhale and lift your hips up while sliding your upper back onto the bench. Your neck should be aligned with the rest of your spine. Other than to check your foot/leg position, you should be looking up at about 10–20 degrees from vertical. Your shins should be vertical and your feet and knees should be aligned with your hips. If your feet are in the wrong position, adjust them before going any farther. **4.** Exhale for a 3 count while lowering your hips with control. As your hips go down, your torso angle must shift from being almost parallel to the floor to almost vertical. Your head moves with the rest of your back, which stays neutral. Don't let your shoulders slide off the bench. **5.** Inhale though your nose then exhale as you quickly and explosively drive your hips back up, squeezing your glutes hard. You should come back up so that your hips are parallel to the floor, with your chest and head facing up. Don't arch your back during this movement—you must maintain neutral spine to avoid injury.

Do 12–15 reps.

Half-Kneeling Hip Flexor Stretch

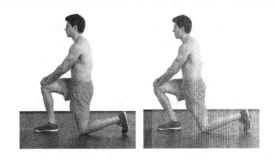

1. Assume the 90/90 position and place both hands on your lead thigh. Tuck your pelvis under so that your hips are under your shoulders and your lower back is flat. You should feel the quads of your rear leg being lightly stretched. **2.** Making sure to keep your pelvis tucked under, push your feet hard into the floor and shift your hips and torso forward an inch or two. The stretch in the trailing quad should be a bit more pronounced. Hold briefly.

Return to start position.

Do 10 reps then switch sides.

Arm Screw

Unlike arm circles where most people just rotate their shoulders with their arms out to the sides this one adds more of a screwing movement and incorporates your entire body. Start off with one arm at a time then move toward doing both arms together and moving the body at the same time.

Level 1: One Arm at a Time

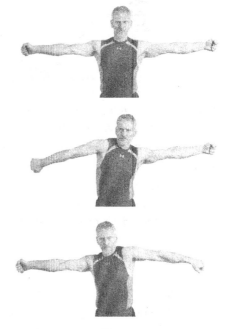

1. Stand with your feet about shoulder-width apart, with your arms out to the sides and parallel to the floor. Your hands should be in fists with palms facing forward. **2.** Without shrugging, suck the shoulder of one arm into its socket. This should make your shoulder rise slightly; your torso may move away from your shoulder a little, which is fine. As your shoulder elevates, rotate the entire arm forward (internal shoulder rotation) so that the thumb side of your fist points down. Extend your shoulder so it drops, keeping your arm parallel to the floor. **3.** Suck your shoulder back into its socket and rotate it backward until the thumb side of your hand points up and you're back at the start position.

Repeat with the other arm.

Perform this movement for 30–45 seconds.

Level 2: Both Arms Together

With this variation, your arms move in opposite directions at the same time.

1. Stand with your feet about shoulder-width apart, with your arms out to the sides and parallel to the floor. Your hands should be in fists with palms facing forward. **2.** Rotate your right arm forward so that the thumb side of your fist points down. Extend your shoulder so it drops, keeping your arm parallel to the floor. Your left arm remains thumb up. **3.** Suck the shoulders of both arms in and rotate your arms so that the thumbs turn over and point in the opposite direction of where they started. You'll probably find your body moving away from the internally rotated shoulder, which is normal.

Reverse the process, sucking in your shoulders and rotating your arms once again.

Perform this movement for 30–45 seconds.

Level 3: One Arm at a Time with Body Movement

1. Stand with your feet about shoulder-width apart, with your arms out to the sides and parallel to the floor. Your hands should be in fists with palms facing forward. **2.** Suck in your right shoulder and rotate your arm forward. At the same time, pivot on your right foot and bend your right knee while turning your knee and body about 45 degrees to the left. Your left leg will also bend but doesn't turn. You're basically moving away from the internal rotation and getting a bit more movement out of your shoulder blade. Think of this movement as wringing out your shoulders as you would a towel. **3.** To return to start position, unwind your torso, hips, and knees so that your feet are back to shoulder-width apart,

hips facing forward. **4.** Repeat with your left arm, bending both knees and pivoting on your left foot until your hips are about 45 degrees to the right.

Return to start position.

Perform this movement for 30–45 seconds.

Level 4: Full Integration

1. Stand with your feet about shoulder-width apart, with your arms out to the sides and parallel to the floor. Your hands should be in fists with palms facing forward. **2.** Suck in your right shoulder and rotate your arm forward. At the same time, pivot on your right foot and bend your right knee while turning your knee and body about 45 degrees to the left. Your left leg will also bend but doesn't turn. **3.** Suck the shoulders into the sockets of both arms at the same time. **4.** Reverse the arm screw on the right and start to internally rotate your left arm. At the same time your body is unwinding, moving back to center and to the right. Your left shoulder is now internally rotated and your right arm is neutral with its thumb up. Your hips are facing 45 degrees to the right. Both knees are bent and your left foot and leg are turned to the right as well.

Keep moving from side to side, smooth and unforced.

Perform this movement for 30–45 seconds.

Forearm Plank

Your goal is to hold this position for a minimum of 2 minutes. Start by going as long as you can, resting briefly, and then doing it again.

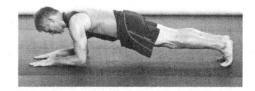

THE POSITION: Place your forearms on the floor parallel to each other; align your elbows under your shoulders. Keep your palms on the floor or place the outer edges of your hands/fists on the floor. Extend your legs behind you like you would for a push-up, keeping your hips in the same plane as your shoulders. Your legs are straight with the balls of the feet actively pushing down and pulling forward. This creates tension in your entire lower body, including your glutes. Actively push down and pull back with your forearms, which creates tension in your upper body.

Make sure your spine is neutral; don't let your back sag or your hips go high or low. Have someone place a piece of PVC on your back. The stick should contact the back of your head, between your shoulder blades and your tailbone, with a slight gap at your lower back.

High Plank

Your goal is at least 2 minutes without losing position.

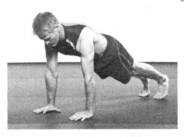

THE POSITION: Get into a push-up position and have someone place a PVC pipe on your back. The points of contact are the back of your head, between your shoulder blades, and your tailbone. Some people extend their hips so that there's a line from the back of their head through their heels, while others keep their hips and shoulders in the same plane. Either is fine, although you have to be careful not to arch your lower back with your hips extended. Hold, maintaining tension throughout

your body, breathing in through your nose and out through your mouth with control.

Bird Dog

Your spine should be neutral and there should be no movement of the torso or hips, shifting to the side, or flexing the spine during the entire sequence. Remember that your foot should not be any higher than your hip, which forces your pelvis to rotate—that's not what we're after.

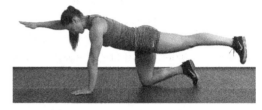

1. Start with your hands under your shoulders and both knees on the floor under your hips. Your thighs should be vertical from the front as well as the sides. Your knees and thighs shouldn't be touching. **2.** Slowly and with control, lift one arm straight out in front of you at shoulder height, fingers pointing straight ahead while also lifting the opposite leg off the floor so that the foot is level with your hip and your toes point straight back. Don't let your hips rotate; they and your shoulders should remain parallel to the floor. Hold this position for 2 full, regular breathing cycles then slowly return your hand and knee to start position.

Switch sides and repeat. Do 8–10 reps per side.

VARIATION: If you can't maintain the one-arm/opposite-leg position, begin by extending one arm at a time. When you can do that with ease and without any shifting, extend one leg at a time, keeping both hands on the floor. Again, there should be no movement except from the leg. When you can do the leg-only version properly, return to doing the full movement.

Half-Kneeling Band Pull

This exercise works on rotational core stability by forcing you not to let the band allow your body to turn or bend when pulling. It's also used to train scapular (shoulder blade) movement and positioning. Your glutes are worked, too, because they're heavily involved in any core function as well as lower-body control during deadlifts, swings, running, and walking. The tempo should be a two-count pull, a one-count hold and a three-count on the extension. Breathe with the movement: Exhale on the pull, pause your breath on the hold, sniff in some air then exhale on the extension.

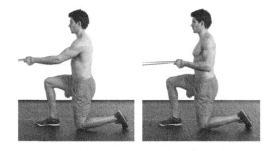

1. Attach a sturdy resistance band to something sturdy without edges or corners. Take the free end of the band and put your right hand through it so that it's on the back of your wrist, then wrap your hand around the band loosely. Don't squeeze the band. If you have a handle, you can use that instead. Step back 2 to 3 feet, depending on the band length, your arm length, and how strong you are. Still holding the band, assume the half-kneeling position with your right knee on the floor. Stay tall; your hips should be under your shoulders. Your right arm should be fully extended with your shoulder in its socket. Your hand should be a little lower than shoulder height and facing across your body. **2.** Pull the band back for a 2 count until it's slightly in front of your ribs at the level of your bottom two ribs. Your elbow will be bent just under 90 degrees and slightly behind your body. **3.**

Slowly extend your arm back to start position for a 3 count, resisting the pull of the band.

Do 12–15 then switch arms.

Half-Kneeling Band Press

This exercise may need a band with less tension than the Half-Kneeling Band Pull since it's harder to push than to pull.

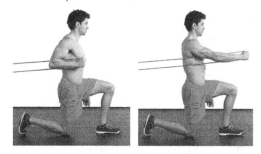

1. Attach a band to something sturdy without edges or corners. Holding the band in your right hand, turn away from the post and go into a half-kneeling position with your right knee on the floor. Take the band and bring it between your arm and your body; the band should be straight behind your armpit. If it's behind your back, it will be angled as it goes under your arm, which makes it even tougher to stay straight. **2.** With the band under your arm, place your hand in the end so it crosses your palm diagonally from the web of your thumb to the heel of your hand below your little finger. **3.** Stay tight, exhale, and extend your arm out to a 3 count. Pause for 2 counts. At the end range, your hand should be about upper chest/shoulder level with your wrist straight and palm facing across your body. Don't overextend your shoulder.

Moving at a 3-count pace, resist the band on the way back in.

Do 12–15 then switch arms.

Pallof Press

The Pallof Press is named after its inventor John Pallof, a physical therapist in Boston, Massachusetts. There are three variations: standing, tall kneeling, and half kneeling, plus overhead movement to all of those. With the exception of the overhead movement, they're all done the same way; there should be no turning of the torso or hips and the line of travel should be perpendicular to your body. You'll need a light to moderate resistance band attached to something sturdy. If you're rotating toward or away from the attachment point or your arms aren't moving in and out in a straight line, there's too much tension on the band. Either move in a little or use a band with less resistance. For all three variations, the band will be at chest level when you're in position. Start with the half-kneeling position then progress over time to tall kneeling and then to standing.

In the half-kneeling position, the knee closest to the attachment point should be down. Make sure you're in proper half-kneeling position (90/90).

In the tall-kneeling version, make sure your knees are hip-width apart. Neither your thighs nor knees should be touching each other.

In standing position, keep the feet hip-width apart or closer. The narrower your base of support, the more your abs have to work.

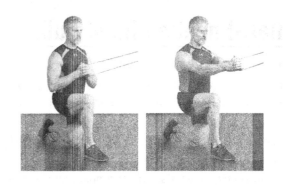

1. Leaving a little slack, hold the band in the fist of the hand nearest the attachment point. Place the other hand around the first. The hand should be in front of your solar plexus with the elbows bent and angled down. You and the band should be perpendicular to the attachment point; your side will be near the post as opposed to facing it.
2. Keeping your core braced, extend both arms in a straight line with no deviation. Your hands should remain in line with your solar plexus throughout the movement. **3.** Slowly bend your elbows and bring the band back to your solar plexus.

Do 12–15 then switch arms.

OVERHEAD-ARMS VARIATION: When your arms are straight, raise them up as high as possible without arching your back, keeping your elbows straight. If you arch your back or start to rotate, you need to stop, lower your arms until they're in line with your solar plexus, bring your arms back in, and start another rep.

ROLLING PATTERNS

Rolling is a fundamental movement that requires the use of the core musculature to execute properly. Rolling is how a baby moves, from face-up to facedown and then to all fours. By learning to roll you'll re-integrate your core with the rest of your body, which will make all of your movements better.

The two basic rolls are the lower-body roll and the upper-body roll. A more advanced version is referred to as the hard roll. The lower-body roll is easier and should be done well before moving to the upper-body roll.

Lower Body Rolling

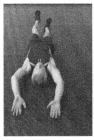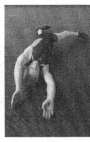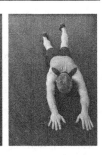

1. Lie on the floor face-up with your arms on the floor above your head and legs straight along the floor. **2.** Keeping your leg straight, raise the foot off the floor and reach with it to the opposite side. As your leg crosses your body, exhale or you'll get stuck. Also look with your eyes in the direction you're rolling. **3.** As your leg completes its reach, your torso should follow and your arms should move last. You should be facedown. **4.** Using the same leg, reach it back behind you and exhale. Don't push off with your arms or your non-working leg. Think about having a rod from the foot of your non-working leg up through your hip and shoulder—that's the axis of rotation. **5.** As your leg finishes its reach, your torso should be rolling and your arms should move last until you're face-up again.

Do 10 rolls to one side then 10 to the other side.

Upper Body Rolling

Although similar to lower body rolling, in this version you initiate with your arms, letting your feet flop over.

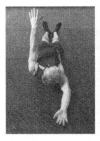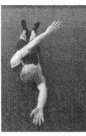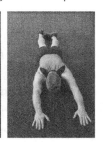

1. Lie face-up with your arms on the floor above your head and legs straight along the floor. **2.** Lift your head and tuck your chin into the shoulder of the side you'll be rolling to. Raise your opposite arm so that it's vertical (if you're rolling to the left, raise your right arm). **3.** Reach your vertical arm across your body and follow with your eyes, exhaling as you go. Keep reaching until your torso is facedown and your lower body flops over. Think of a rod from the heel of your foot through your shoulder of the side you're rolling toward. Your legs stay straight at all times; avoid folding at the hips or waist. Don't push off with either leg or the non-working arm. **4.** From the facedown position, reach back with the same arm you started with and look back behind you with your head and eyes. Keep reaching behind you and exhale as you come over your side. **5.** As you go face-up, your torso will be face-up first, followed by your hips. Your legs should flop over.

INDEX

G

Grip: for clean, 83–84; for jerk, 108; for snatch, 117

H

Half-kneeling position, 27

Halting Deadlift (snatch), 128–29

Hand placement: for clean, 83–84; for jerk, 108; for snatch, 117

Hang Clean, 83, 96–97

Hang position, 26; for clean, 83, 86; for snatch, 118

Hang Power Clean, 94–95

Hang Power Snatch, 130–31

Hang Snatch, 136–37

Hang Snatch & Squat, 135

High pull (clean), 83, 89–90

Hip mobility assessment, 32–33, 34

Hook grip, for clean, 83–84

Hurdle Step (hip mobility/core stability assessment), 32

Hydration, 25

Hypertrophy training, 9

Hyponatremia, 25

I

Intermediate workout program, 55–66

J

Jerk, 12, 107–16; Power Jerk from Behind the Neck, 113; Power Jerk in Front of the Neck, 114; practice exercises, 107; Press, 109; Press from Behind the Neck, 108; Push Press, 111–12; Push Press from Behind the Neck, 110; Split Jerk, 115–16; terminology, 107–108

Jerk blocks/boxes, for weightlifting, 18

K

Kettlebell rack position, 26

Knee dip, for jerk, 108

Knurling, of barbell, 17

L

Lacrosse balls, and SMFR, 19, 39

Lifting area. *See* Platform

Lifting chalk. *See* Chalk

Lifting straps, 19

"Lifting weights," 12

Lifts, 81–140; clean, 12, 13, 82–106; jerk, 12, 107–16; missed, 21; snatches, 13, 117–40

Lunge (hip mobility assessment), 32–33

M

Massage sticks, 19

Medical clearance, 20

Missed lifts, escaping, 21

Muscle Clean, 92

Muscle High Pull (clean), 87–88

Muscle Snatch, 123

N

Needle bearings, 16–17

Neutral spine assessment, 35–36

90/90 position (half-kneeling position), 27

Nutrition, 22–25

O

Oiling, of barbell, 17

Olympic weightlifting, 12–13; basic positions, 26–27; and CrossFit, 8, 14–15; equipment, 16–19; exercises, 141–85; history, 10–11; lifts, 81–140; and nutrition, 22–25; safety, 9, 20–21; self-assessment tests, 28–36, 40–41; terminology, 16–19, 83–84, 107–108, 117–18; vs. bodybuilding, 9; workout programs, 38–80

1 rep max (1RM), 67, 68

Overhand grip, for clean, 83

Overhead Squat: shoulder assessment, 30; snatch (with barbell), 119–20

Straps, for weightlifting, 19
Sugary foods, 24–25

T

Tall-kneeling position, 27
Tennis balls, and SMFR, 19, 39
Terminology, 16–19, 83–84, 107–108, 117–18
Trigger points, 19, 39
Trunk Stability Push-Up (TSPU), 35
Two-Phase Snatch, 132

V

Vegetables, 24

W

Warming up, 38–39; dynamic warm-ups, 41. *See also*
    specific programs
Water, 25
Weightlifting. *See* Olympic weightlifting
Workout programs, 38–80; Phase I: Beginner Program,
    43–54; Phase II: Intermediate Program, 55–66;
    Phase III: Advanced Program, 67–80; workout key,
    42

INDEX OF EXERCISES AND ASSISTANCE LIFTS

ACKNOWLEDGMENTS

I'd like to thank my wife, Cheryl, for being so supportive. I'd also like to thank all of my current and past clients, without whom I wouldn't be where I am today. A huge shout out to Bernadett Temesi for helping me run the gym, especially when I need to travel! Thanks to Jamie Hale. If it weren't for him, I would've never been asked to write *Spartan Warrior Workout* and my other books. Last but not least, thanks to Claire Chun and Lily Chou of Ulysses Press for putting up with me and cleaning up my writing. It's always a pleasure to work with you!

ABOUT THE AUTHOR

DAVE RANDOLPH, author of *Spartan Warrior Workout*, *The Ultimate Kettlebell Workbook*, and *Action Movie Hero Workouts*, has been involved in martial arts since 1989, earning the rank of Master, 6th-degree black belt, in 2005. Through his martial arts training and teaching, Dave became interested in teaching fitness to more than just martial artists. In 2002, he became certified as a kettlebell instructor under Pavel Tsatsouline, who brought kettlebells into the mainstream around 1998. In 2007, he began teaching fitness at the only full-time kettlebell-centric gym in Louisville, Kentucky. Since then, Dave's unique methods have helped thousands of people become healthier and fitter.

Dave has studied kettlebells under several highly regarded kettlebell instructors and is constantly seeking to learn from the best in all fields in order to improve himself and what he teaches. By integrating joint mobility, strength, agility, flexibility, and coordination, Dave's constantly evolving IronBody Fitness shows people how to elevate their health, fitness levels, and quality of life. He's currently a Certified Kettlebell Teacher (CKT) Level II with the International Kettlebell and Fitness Federation (IKFF) and competes in kettlebell sport. He also trains in Filipino martial arts.

In 2007, Dave became a Level 1 CrossFit affiliate and has trained Olympic lifting under Jamie Hale in Winchester, Kentucky. The next year Dave became a Certified FMS practitioner and uses the FMS screens on all his clients to make sure they're doing what they need to train safely.

If you'd like Dave to teach kettlebells in your area, or if you're a fitness professional looking to become a top-notch certified kettlebell instructor, visit Dave's website, www.iron-body.com, or kbuniversity.com.

Made in the USA
Monee, IL
27 January 2025

11047589R00109